THE CHILD, HIS "ILLNESS,"
AND THE OTHERS

MAUD MANNONI

THE CHILD, HIS "ILLNESS," AND THE OTHERS

Translated from the French

PANTHEON BOOKS

A Division of Random House, New York

FOR BRUNO

Preface to the English-Language Edition

This work springs from a revaluation of accepted ideas in psychoanalysis. It is an attempt to resume contact with Freud's thought in all its rigor, for its impact has become weakened with the passage of time, as the first shock waves caused by the discovery of psychoanalysis have died down.

Stress is laid throughout this book not so much on *intersubjective* relations as on *language*—the framework the child enters at birth, but one shaped long before it.

I emphasize that which in the parents' discourse will or will not allow the child to accede to words of his own. Psychoanalysis can not isolate the "sick" child's symptom from the parents' words. Child and parents should not be split into separate, watertight compartments, nor should the parents be psychoanalyzed for their child's "good." What is needed is to evoke, beyond the wall of language, a locus of truth, truth of a knowledge which the child suppresses in his parents by his symptom.

There is a good deal of talk about the Oedipus complex, as if it were an "illness," and as if the analyst's main job were to correct or not to correct this particular one. Clinically, it is clear that the Oedipus complex (the introduction of a Symbolic order) is above all the expression of an unsolved problem of the parents in regard to their own parents, of which the child, by his symptom, has become the representative signifier.

As soon as the psychoanalytic act gets under way the analyst has a place in the collective discourse. He does not stand outside it as an impartial observer, but is at the very heart of the words brought to him by the child and his family. In the established transference situation he occupies a place sometimes on the Real level, sometimes on the Imaginary level (he is then the other of the patient, whose ego is alienated in the image of other people or, indeed, he is the other, who supports the partial object), sometimes on the Symbolic level (he is then the Other, "the locus where the 'I' is formed which speaks to the one who hears" [Jacques Lacan]).

The truth which emerges in an analysis is always the action on the living being of an action of the *Symbolic*. In this perspective, the truth becomes the cause of the subject of the unconscious, of the subject which is revealed in the analysand's words and which is not the classic subject generally referred to.

Thus, the psychoanalyst studies man not as a being of need but as a being of *desire*. For desire to emerge from need, it must be formulated in a demand. This can only be expressed in the order of language. Man's drama is inscribed in a sort of basic imbalance between the desire and its object. Analysis is at grips with this dilemma. It unveils for the subject the falsehood in which he had become lost with the complicity of an other, a half truth-half falsehood the present form of which is his symptom. The symptom is a masked word or lost words which must be reintegrated with the past history of the speaking subject. The assumption of a truth (through anxiety about death and castration) is achieved in the Symbolic order and not in the Real or Imaginary order.

Man's desire to manifest himself is marked by a stamp which is everything Lacan designates by the name of the paternal metaphor (a world of objects taken in the order of signifiers). The paternal metaphor has nothing to do with the reality of a "strong" or "weak" father but with his presence in what he symbolizes in the mother's words. Analysts are too inclined to allow themselves to become fascinated by the real figures of the parents, who may be well or ill assorted; some analysts even go so far as to adjure a father to be more manly or a mother to be more tender. All such attempts at normalization let slip the effects of truth which have to be disentangled from the family drama, in order to restore meaning to the subject (who has often been robbed of all words of his own).

Throughout his writings, Lacan distinguishes the "I" of the subject from his ego; he stresses the fact that the ego is the locus of all Imaginary identifications, the locus of all snares and all failures of recognition.

The subject has his words stolen by an ego who is there in order not to hear him. Only the Symbolic dimension (the third element which intervenes in the dual relation of the child to the mother) can enable the subject to disentangle his words from all the snares and fascinations in which he has been lost at certain stages of his existence—to disengage them too from all the struggles for face or struggles to the death which are specific to dual situations.

The importance which I attach to the different orders (the Real, the Imaginary, and the Symbolic) constitutes the main thread of this book. In the chapter on transference, I analyze the misunderstandings and misconceptions which occur for want of the analyst's having tracked down on what level the one who was speaking was situated (the stake is not the same, if the patient, in the Imaginary order, is speaking to an other who is himself or if he is appealing, in the Symbolic order, to the Other in order that meaning may be restored to him).

Our view of a "sick" person is moreover impeded by the idea we have of him. If the patient presents himself to us behind a mask, we, for our part, put up a screen which distorts our relation to the other. (I have attempted to develop this point at length in my book *L'Enfant arriéré et sa mère* [The Retarded Child and His Mother].) In our relation to the other, our own view of the world intervenes. This is why we must take care not to raise this view to dogma or ideology; if we do, we shall become the accomplices of the representatives of order and of the Church, masking a form of dishonesty behind an alleged objectivity.[1]

I make many references to Melanie Klein; I have, however, taken her theory of "good" and "bad" objects out of a sort of objectified materiality in which it had become bogged down. The Kleinian theory, as Lacan has shown, can be articulated in terms of signifiers; the entire dialectic of good and bad objects are signs which reveal how the subject is in a dilemma as soon as he becomes the subject of desire, for want of being able to situate himself with regard to an object which is simultaneously good and bad.

If, in the clinical field, I have given proof of originality, daring, and independence, I owe everything in the field of theory to my master, Jacques Lacan.[2]

In my accounts of the analysis of psychotics, I show how only a structural approach makes it possible to discern what is in play in a psychosis. I emphasize that psychosis cannot be approached correctly unless all development theories are discarded—but this brings us back to our starting point, stripping the veil from the myths which we have built up to defend ourselves against "mental illness," indeed against all challenges from the unconscious which we must face when we allow ourselves to listen to that vast symptomatic utterance which includes the child, his "illness," his parents, and ourselves.

Paris   M.M.
September, 1968

---

[1] J. Lacan, "La Science et la vérité," in *Écrits* (Paris, Seuil, 1966). "To say that the subject on which we work in psychoanalysis can only be the subject of science may be considered a paradox. It is nevertheless at this point that a dividing line should be drawn, in default of which everything becomes mixed up and dishonesty begins which will moreover be called objectivity. In our position of subject, we are always responsible. Any attempt to incarnate the subject in more reality is errant—always fruitful in error and as such faulty as it is to incarnate it in the man, who there comes back to the child. For the man will be the primitive and that will falsify the whole primal process while the child will play the part of underdeveloped man and that will mask the truth of what is happening during original childhood."

[2] His first work was on the "mirror-phase," a statement of what was to be later introduced under the name of structure (and its articulation with the Symbolic, the Real, and the Imaginary).

Acknowledgments

Much of the material in this book originally formed the subject of lectures at the universities of Strasbourg, Louvain, Brussels, and Rome, under the auspices of Professors Israel, Schotte, Vergote, de Waelhens, Sivadon and Bollea.

My thanks are due to P. Aulagnier, M.-C. Boons, J. Barmont, F. Dolto, M. Drazien, E. Gasquères, L. Irigaray, Ch. Melman, L. Mélèse, G. Michaud, D. Lambert, J. Oury, M. Safouan, J.-P. Sichel, C. Simatos, A.-L. Stern, R. Tostain, and P. Rufenacht for their collaboration in teamwork on the problems of an Externat médico-pédagogique.

Thanks are also due to Professor Anthony Wilden, of the University of California at San Diego, and to the Johns Hopkins Press for their kind permission to use, in the glossary of the present book, material from *The Language of the Self* (1968), Professor Wilden's book on Jacques Lacan's "Discours de Rome."

I am indebted, in matters of theory, to the thought of Jacques Lacan. I also acknowledge the help of my husband and of Colette Audry who both gave a critical hearing to these pages.

M. M.

A Note on the Translation

The author is a follower of Jacques Lacan and uses his specialized vocabulary. To assist readers in following Lacan's theories, this translation generally employs the terminology worked out by Professor Anthony Wilden of the University of California for his translation of and commentary on Lacan's "Discours de Rome," *The Language of the Self: The Function of Language in Psychoanalysis,* published in 1968 by the Johns Hopkins Press.

For the English-speaking reader who may not be familiar with Lacan's theories and vocabulary, the author has supplied a short discussion of Lacan's ideas, followed by a glossary of the principal words in his terminology (see pages 262–80).

"We have really understood when we become part of what has been said to us."

MARTIN HEIDEGGER

Contents

THE CHILD, HIS "ILLNESS,"
AND THE OTHERS

THE PSYCHOANALYSIS OF CHILDREN SINCE FREUD

The psychoanalysis of children is psychoanalysis in its purest form. That was Freud's conviction in 1909 when he was treating a five-year-old child afflicted with a phobic neurosis.[1] The adaptation of the technique to the special situation that approaching a child conveys to the adult leaves open the entire field in which the analyst functions—the field of language (even when the child does not yet speak). Communication involves parents, child, and analyst; it is a collective process centering around the child's symptom. The disorder *which is spoken about* is reifiable in the person of the child, but the parental complaint, if its subject is the real child, also reveals by its implications the adult's conception of childhood. Society confers a special status on the child by expecting him, all unknowing, to fulfill the future of the adult. It is the child's task to make good the parents' failures, to make their lost dreams come true. The complaints of parents about their offspring thus refer us first of all to their own problems. The same characteristic emerges in analysis when the adult tells us about his own past. What he

---

[1] S. Freud, "Analysis of a Phobia in a Five-Year-Old Boy" in Standard Edition of the *Complete Psychological Works,* trans. and ed. J. Strachey (London, Hogarth Press, 1966), Vol. X.

describes is not so much a reality experienced as a dream betrayed.

In the beginning of psychoanalysis, childhood was presented in the recollection of adults only in the sense of repressed memories. What was at issue was not so much the real past as the way it was situated in a certain perspective; in reconstructing his childhood the subject reorganized the past according to his desire, like a small child at play who reorganizes his present or past world to suit his fancy. Words surge forth to make contact with a real or imaginary adult—indeed, an imaginary companion. In psychoanalysis, the verbal accounts of children as well as of adults refer us not so much to realities as to worlds of desires and dreams.

As early as 1918, this truth was lost sight of by Hug-Hellmuth, the first analyst who dealt with children, and thus, from the beginning, analysis developed in two opposite directions. In one, the discoveries of Freud were retained intact (particularly, the Oedipus complex and transference); in the other, they were disregarded in order to change a reality: the child becomes the prop of the good intentions that adults sustain in his behalf.

For that reason, the psychoanalyst confronted with the child takes part in the treatment with his own prejudices (his countertransference). Even before Freud's time, the doctor did not want to understand what the child was indicating to him, not only through the symptom, but even by endeavoring to put it into words. Freud offers us the example of a medical thesis presented in 1881 by one Dr. Debacker,[2] which ignored in its conclusions all the clinical data

---

[2] See S. Freud, *The Interpretation of Dreams* (London, Allen & Unwin, 1954), p. 585. Freud quotes the medical thesis put forth in 1881 by Debacker. It deals with a boy of thirteen who had had disturbed nights, night terrors, and hallucinations since the age of eleven. The Devil appeared to him in dreams, alone or in the company of others, and shouted, "Now we've got you, now we've got you." The child smelled pitch and brimstone and his skin seemed to him to be burned by flames. He cried out, "No, it's not me, it's not me, I've not done anything," or else, "Leave me alone, leave me alone, I won't do it again." He refused to get undressed for fear of being consumed by the flames. Adults sent the child into the country for a year and a half. He returned, having recovered but still remembering his past fears. On reaching puberty, he gave the following explanation of his "illness": "I did not dare admit it, but I was continually having prickly feelings and

recorded in observation. Instead of data, Debacker postulated medical theories that had no connection with what the patient had said. This attitude (which can be found in other guises today) led Freud to denounce "pseudoscience" as the opposite of true research. In his thesis, Debacker proposed a diagnosis of cerebral anemia (which supposedly caused the demonomanic hallucinations of the child), but his diagnosis had very little connection with the actual clinical history. Debacker paid no attention to the patient's words, although he had recorded them in his notes. An uninitiated person, says Freud, would have done better; he would have been struck by the words uttered by the boy who was in the grip of acute persecution anxiety. The key to his somatic disorder was given by the boy the day he got better, and the cure occurred as soon as he was able to verbalize the meaning of his "illness"—indicating in words what the symptom had kept veiled. It was by the indirect means of hallucinatory accusations that the child got out the "first words," namely, the guilt-laden confession of having masturbated. Hallucinated or accusatory words in delusions are usually words that have been heard but forgotten, which leave their trace at the level of the symptom. In the course of an analysis, it is possible to detect the imprint of words (said or unsaid) on the soma.[3] In this particular case, the boy acted as his own physician.

As a clinician, Freud listened first to what the symptom was telling him; it is the only method that makes it possible to adopt an analytic attitude toward neurosis, especially child neurosis. Subsequently, Freud's researches continued in two different directions;

---

overexcitement in my parts; in the end it got on my nerves so much that I often thought of jumping out of the dormitory window." Freud emphasized the link between the various symptoms and the repressed desire to masturbate: "The fear of punishment, indeed the struggle against a guilt-laden desire was transformed, according to him, into anxiety." Debacker had simply diagnosed it as a cerebral disorder.

[3] Here "word" (parole) is used in the sense of something said or unsaid, which has left its imprint or the absence of which has left its imprint on the subject hearing it. This imprint is reproduced in the symptom, which may be psychological or somatic.

on the one hand, he delved deeper into the meaning of the symptom, which he conceived as "word," [4] yet on the other hand, a belief (non-scientific) in the physiologic origin of psychic disorders caused him to direct his attention to the importance of trauma in the genesis of neuroses (1896). Nevertheless, he soon discovered by analyzing hysterics that the childhood they were talking about was not always their real childhood, and that the traumas they were alluding to might well have been fictitious. He found that words, even lies, constituted in themselves the truth of the subject; what was said had to be integrated with the discourse of the unconscious. Childhood memories and "traumas" assume meaning when they are situated in relation to the *desire* of the subject.

Thus, these discoveries do not refer us back to a real childhood or to the history of an individual development, but to the language of the unconscious. Nevertheless, Freudian ideas have been stretched sometimes in the quest for psychophysical parallelism. It was thought that the "maturation" process of the child could be better understood in this way. Certain analysts (Hug-Hellmuth, the Vienna school, the Zurich school) thought that Freud's and Abraham's theory of stages provided medical bases for a conception of pedagogy, indeed for a form of psychoanalysis conceived essentially as educational (Anna Freud). The child, say the educationalists, is susceptible to measures of conditioning or training, and the possibilities of adapting the theory in reality have been explored by a long line of researchers from Pfister through Pavlov to Piaget. But, if the description of stages (oral, anal, genital) occupies an important place in the works of Abraham, it is because he regards them primarily as positions successively occupied by the subject confronted by desire in a fantasy relationship to an object. It was in this sense, following the path taken by Abraham, that Melanie

---

[4] Freud assumed that it was in obedience to strict laws that effects of the displacement or condensation mechanism appeared in the words of the subject. He utilized the decoding of unconscious speech in *The Interpretation of Dreams* and in the analysis of the Rat Man. We are thus introduced to the idea of reading the symptom (obsessional or hysterical) that the subject presents.

Klein pursued her inquiries. She describes anxiety *situations* occurring at such and such a stage in the history of the subject—a subject *marked* by the effect produced by certain events in his life, above all, by words, which he tries to forget, cancel, or put into effect, depending on whether they refer him back to the power of a particular family myth.

Freud [5] looked to child analysis for confirmation of his theories. He appreciated the richness of observation it afforded, and it was for this reason that the work of Hug-Hellmuth on infantile sexuality caught his attention. Years later, the observations of Anna Freud and Dorothy Burlingham at the Hampstead War Nursery made a valuable contribution to Freud's hypotheses by confirming the irreversible effects of certain conditions of life. Nevertheless, the possibility of treating serious cases remained doubtful for a long time. Psychoanalysts accented the scientific validity of facts derived from experiment and observation, confirming Freud's conceptions, but they displayed a certain resistance to making use of these discoveries in treatment; thus, Hug-Hellmuth practiced analysis without taking repression into account, that is, without touching on the Oedipal problem. Yet, Freud himself showed as early as 1909 that his discoveries could be utilized in actually treating children. At that time, he was treating the father of a little boy of five, Hans, who himself was suffering from phobic anxiety. Freud agreed to see the boy on various occasions, although he assigned to the father the role of observer and intermediary; the father's task was to record the daily doings and sayings of his son, and Freud undertook to reveal their meaning to the father who was to convey it to Hans.

The child very quickly put "Professor Freud" in the place of a symbolic Father, and in the words that came from that locus he

---

[5] S. Freud, "On the History of the Psycho-Analytic Movement" in Standard Edition of the *Complete Psychological Works,* trans. and ed. J. Strachey (London, Hogarth Press, 1966), Vol. XIV, p. 55. As early as 1914, Freud insisted on the fact that any analysis, and especially any analysis of children, if properly conducted, makes it possible to demonstrate the correctness of the analyst's theoretical orientation.

was trying to attain the truth of his desire. Hans was conscious enough of the Oedipal drama he was living through, and he was embarrassed by the idea that the adult did not want him to know what he already knew (the mysteries of procreation, etc.). Freud situated Hans's Oedipal jealousy in a story he told him and thereby introduced a myth which was then taken up by Hans in various guises throughout the treatment. Hans felt that he got hold of a guiding thread. Next, by means of certain terms,[6] and through castration fantasies, he succeeded in reorganizing his Oedipal problem; it was then that he got better. Freud thus proved the efficacy of bringing unconscious tendencies to the conscious level.

Child psychoanalysis was demonstrated as being practicable. The analysis of Hans became the first example of its kind by proving that interpretation with a child was possible. Since Freud was also the analyst of Hans's father, he could not prevent the treatment of the child from increasing the incompatibility of the parents; the fantasy effects of the problems of the parents had scarcely been studied. Hans's father, with his child, was linked to Freud on the Imaginary plane. They competed with each other in what they told "Professor Freud." The interest of Hans switched from the women at home to those in Freud's house. The boy's mother, without being aware of it, felt excluded and was constantly intervening with words which had the effect of undoing Freud's work. As Hans could not rely on his mother, the maid came to play the part of female substitute for him, because he could talk to her about sex without shocking her. Struggling with difficulties, which she had to overcome unaided, Hans's mother fell back on her daughter, and took a woman friend into her confidence. In her world there was no longer any place for a man's words, and we know that later on she left her family and lived alone, without a man. A divorce might have been avoided if Freud had paid greater heed to the mother's grievances; analysis "stole" first her husband from her and then her son, and she found only a woman friend (who knew nothing about

6 These terms were signifiers such as the Name of the Father, the phallus, etc.

8

analytic matters) to confide in. Both parents fell into a situation of regressive homosexuality; it was their way of participating in the questions brought to the surface by Hans. The dialogue between Freud and Hans provided a place where the fantasies of all the adults converged, in which Hans represented the adult desire.[7]

It was therefore the reality of the child they were pursuing through various medical and educational perspectives, particularly under the influence of Pfister. But, in the analysis of Little Hans, Freud clearly pinpointed the place occupied by the child in his mother's fantasy.[8] When we reread the text, we are struck by the manner in which Hans's questions produced a reaction in the unconscious of the adults. The child was the support for the sexual problem which the parents could not face. He unmasked things they had hoped to keep hidden, and he thereby put his parents in an awkward situation (the servant whose sex life was apparently satisfactory was much less embarrassed). It is remarkable to see to what extent the child, by his mere presence, brought into play not so much the relationship of his parents to himself as the relationship of each parent to his own problems—to the point where their sex life finally broke down. But the situation confronting the analyst is alien to any interpersonal relationship because at bottom it is a matter of the relation of the subject to his desire. This relation was further complicated in the case of Hans in the sense that he had to cut across the field of parental desire to attain the truth of his own desire, and in that his mother denied him access to it by opposing his unconscious wish[9] that he become phallic, forever the

[7] The father's desire for Freud and the theoretical interest of the case for Freud's research.

[8] By rejecting her son in reality (and subsequently all men), the mother indicated that she found it impossible to give up the Imaginary object which her son, as phallic substitute, represented for her.

[9] *Wish* (*Wunsch*): Freud distinguishes, in *The Interpretation of Dreams,* between "desire" and "inclination"; desire is contrasted with need and reveals what is deceptive in inclination. He shows that the wish in a dream can refer to a *desire* which finds expression in deceptive joking or mystifying speech. He takes as an example the dream of a hysteric associated with a wish for caviar; he shows us

9

subject of her admiring gaze. She refused him his masculinity, and made it very clear to him in *words,* by giving him to understand that she did not want any man. It was from the moment that she uttered these words that Hans found himself unable to express what he needed to articulate in order to get out of the Oedipal stage. Later, by forging the instrument of his own cure—his myths —Hans achieved independence; the mother, unfortunately, responded to it by "abandoning" him in reality. Although at that stage Freud could not foresee all the complications of the situation in which his patient had involved him, he nevertheless gives us a remarkably precise description of it. By becoming the analyst of father and son without listening to the mother's words, Freud became a third party between father and mother and satisfied (more completely than he had intended) the fantasies of his patient. He was unable to help the mother to put up with a situation which she did not understand, and its effects were transferred to an increasingly marked hostility towards men.

It took time for analysts to understand where the importance of Freud's contribution to child psychoanalysis lay. It seemed to them that they could not carry out a proper analytic investigation with a child, because the very memories of childhood constituted the objective of their work with adults—or so they thought. He saw in it the origin of the unreasoning fear some children have of the parent of the same sex, which is internalized as a threat and then projected to the external world which is thereupon felt to be menacing. Starting with these neglected ideas, Melanie Klein found new recognition points[10] to be applied in working with psychotic children, which are well known today. The sources of her formulations lay

---

that this wish to have caviar sends the dreamer back by the interplay of displacements to the desire to have an unfulfilled desire. Lacan connects desire with the imprint of language; he makes it the specificity of the Freudian unconscious.

[10] Melanie Klein describes how the child, at the zenith of the Oedipus complex, projects his aggression on the parent who becomes an introjected ogre in his fantasy and as such forms his superego. She distinguishes between two important phases in the life of the child: the paranoid-schizoid position, which she places in the first months of life, characterized by a persecution anxiety, and the depressive position, culminating in the middle of the first year. The typical depressive anxiety seems

in the work of her teacher Karl Abraham[11] and of Freud, who had dealt with Abraham's discoveries in his *Mourning and Melancholia*. Melanie Klein does not concern herself with behavior from the viewpoint of reality, and she breaks with the criteria of adjustment and educability that Anna Freud adopted as guidelines. For her, the matter to be studied lay in the fantasy aspect of the mother-child link in a dual situation, and she highlights the fierceness of the destructive tension that accompanies the love drive. This idea had been touched on by Abraham and Freud; they had stressed the importance of the play of opposites in the conception of the object relationship, i.e., the paradoxical equivalence of apparently opposite expressions—good-bad, give-receive, preserve-destroy.

Melanie Klein evolved these ideas in her study on the sense of guilt in children.[12] She worked on the idea of ambivalence, that is, the presence of an aggressive intention in all love drives. The unconscious situation, which the child fails to recognize, impels him in certain states of crisis to attempt to repair an Imaginary injury he thinks he has inflicted on his mother. These conceptions make it possible to understand what takes place in certain psychotic conditions where the subject struggles with ideas of persecution, i.e., with murderous or suicidal intentions that lead him to compulsive self-defense against his own aggressive projection (against a danger non-existent in reality). In Melanie Klein's view, the child divides the world into "good" and "bad" objects. He attributes to them a protective or aggressive role, alternately, against a danger which he places sometimes inside and sometimes outside himself.

Lacan[13] has sought to define more closely the impact of Kleinian

---

to result from a kind of synthesis by the subject who is seeking to escape from a situation of alternatives without an outlet (in Kleinian language, good and bad objects). The pathological reactions take the form of manic defenses, except where the subject reverts to an earlier persecutory situation.

[11] G. Rosolato and D. Widlöcher, "Karl Abraham: Lecture de son oeuvre," *La Psychanalyse,* Vol. IV (1958).

[12] D. W. Winnicott, "Psychoanalysis and the Sense of Guilt" in *The Maturational Processes and the Facilitating Environment* (New York, International Universities Press; London, Hogarth Press, 1965).

[13] J. Lacan, in seminars, January 28, 1959, June 17, 1959 (unpublished).

ideas; he translates the dialectics of good and bad objects into the language of *desire,* and links it to the unconscious doubletalk of which Freud speaks (in which the "How handsome he is" of the mother's actual words is superimposed on the "Let him die" of her repressed words). Thus, according to him, the Kleinian bad object is situated in the Imaginary plane between the two chains of overt and repressed speech. Melanie Klein's work would gain by being elaborated in the field of words. It has been all too often misdirected to an alleged reality derived from actual experience. She has been consistently weighed down in her writing by the influence of behaviorism. Yet, in spite of the awkward exposition, we can glimpse the pattern that guided her in her clinical work, namely the effects of the interplay of signifiers on the child.

Laing starts from a point postulated by Ludwig Binswanger.[14] Binswanger has highlighted the existential drama of the patient by showing how the symptom is directed to another, and develops with and for another. Laing[15] himself sees the child's position not so much in terms of an interpersonal relationship as in those of the mother's fantasy. He seeks to define the concept of identity in a subject, based on clinical cases as we shall see in the following example.

The case was that of a four-year-old boy called Brian who was taken by his mother to meet a couple who were to adopt him. The mother kissed her child, burst into tears, and ran out without a word. Brian never saw her again. The child was utterly confused; he didn't want the couple as his new parents. They tried to establish themselves for him by saying, "You are our son." But the child would not accept it. He became difficult and, gradually, completely maladjusted.

Brian no longer knew *who he was,* Laing explains. His first iden-

14 Binswanger was first to introduce psychoanalysis in a psychiatric clinic, sometime before 1920. He sought to restructure the traditional hospital setup and provide living conditions for the psychiatric patient that approached normal.

15 R. D. Laing, *The Self and Others,* 2nd ed. (New York, Pantheon Books; London, Tavistock, 1969).

tity was that of being the son of his mother. When his mother went away, he awaited her return to be sure again who he was. During her absence he was simply one who was waiting—he could not be anything else. But, though Brian no longer knew who he was, he did know *what he was:* he was wicked because his mother had got rid of him. In a lengthy analysis Laing demonstrates that it was on the basis of this conviction that the child, traumatized by having been abandoned, built his life. "Since I am bad, there is nothing else to be but bad," Brian explained later.

Although Laing suspected the importance of the part played by the child in the fantasy of the mother, he has nevertheless not made full use of it in his research. It should be possible therefore to develop this study more fully.

Between the *who am I* and the *what I am* posited by Brian, there is a split, the importance of which Laing may not have sufficiently appreciated. In the past which linked Brian to his mother, he had her words that defined him as her son. Although he had lost her, Brian retained in himself these past references which placed him in a specific line of descent. The traumatic experience was the means by which the child found himself flung into another line of descent without a word of explanation. That was the starting point of the drama. He then had to build his life on the basis of words that had been foreclosed. "You are our son," said his adopted parents, but the mother rendered the transition impossible by never having indicated to him in words that he was no longer her child. Thereafter Brian demonstrated how bad he was, conforming to what his new parents were saying about him. In other words, while making a clean sweep of the past in real life, the adults forgot the words of the past which remained inscribed in the child's unconscious and continued to produce effects at the level of the symptom. The traumatic situation can be understood only by reference to the mother's doubletalk (even before abandoning him the mother's words must have referred the child to a form of curse or hate at one of their levels).

In another study, Laing cites a range of maternal modes of discourse in which one can see how a schizogenic situation may be created in the child. The studies have the merit of calling into question matters that were previously developed in terms of environment. It is illuminating to read about the childhood of schizophrenics who have grown up in a crossfire of contradictory orders from their earliest years. Since each demand of the mother has a double in her desire to the contrary, the only choice left to the child is submission to the mother's wish that he not be born to desire.

These researches are related to the analytic line adopted by various theorists in an effort to return to the source of Freudian inspiration, which is none other than a return to the study of unconscious discourse. Child psychoanalysis has repeatedly fallen into traps of educationalist, social, or moral ideology. We have seen how two lines of thought have coexisted from the outset; although the child is sometimes studied as a real object, he is also perceived in the locus where he appears in adult discourse, and his childhood is then transposed into the world of fantasy. The problem recurs every time one confronts a child; the analyst is faced with his own representation of childhood, and the weight of his unconscious motivation will make itself felt in the manner in which he handles the treatment. The child and his family arouse the most primitive fears, defenses, and anxiety in the analyst—he is always being forced into a field where everyone is brought face to face with the problem of desire, death, and the Law.

When Freud [16] talks about the place of parents in the childhood of the subject, he stresses that their real qualities are much less important than what has marked them in their own childhood. Erik Erikson[17] attributes the subject's dependence on the "imprint" [18] to the unconscious part played by different types of ego-ideal, i.e., the catchwords that prevailed in various periods of family life. Thus

16 S. Freud, *An Outline of Psychoanalysis,* in Standard Edition, Vol. XXIII.

17 E. H. Erikson, *Childhood and Society,* 2nd ed. (New York, Norton, 1964; London, Penguin Books, 1965).

18 Lacan approaches this problem as the relation of the subject to the signifier.

the idea is confirmed that conflicts fasten around disseminated words; they conceal the subject's fear of discovering the fragility of his ideal identity. An insight into the resistance arising from the conflict of the ego-ideal makes it possible to lay bare a still more primal core, "the fear of losing hard-won identities." This is certainly one of Erikson's most original points. He places identity in a historical context. Unlike Laing, Erikson is of the opinion that the child develops a separate identity very early—separate from that of his parents—which he sometimes renounces through anxiety, substituting blind identifications. The child can accept parental deprivation if an image beyond that of the real parent can be brought into play in treatment. (Lacan uses the expression "Symbolic dimension" to describe this conception.) Thus Erikson's researches are linked to the work of the Kleinian school; he is careful to show that it is possible to use with children a style of analysis related to adult analysis, and he insists on the importance of the *unsaid* in the constitution of the symptom, following Freud's example toward the study of symptomatic discourse.

We have seen that since Freud's time a movement has grown to save analysis from the organic and pedagogic blind alleys where it was floundering. The clinical approach has been influenced by a succession of theoretical positions. Differences in levels of interpretation have come to light; in particular, technique stresses either play or words as means of expression. However, this sort of distinction ought to be abandoned, because in an analysis play must be understood not on the level of an experience that has been lived (with cathartic effects as in psychodrama), but as one of the elements or incidents of the discourse going on. Freud's observations on this point can be read in this perspective.

It was in 1908 [19] that Freud first spoke of the child's play. He compared it to poetic creation. The child at play, he tells us, creates a world of his own, or rather rearranges the things of his world in a new way that pleases him. In 1920,[20] Freud became interested in the

[19] S. Freud, "The Poet and Daydreaming," in Standard Edition, Vol. IX.
[20] S. Freud, *Beyond the Pleasure Principle,* in Standard Edition, Vol. XVIII.

problem raised in neuroses by the repetition principle. It seemed to him that play activities followed the same principle. The child is endeavoring in his play to master unpleasant experiences, that is, to reproduce a situation that had been too much for him originally. By repeating it, the subject sets his seal on it, *he does over what has been done to him*. Freud makes an observation here which was to be of outstanding importance. He describes an eighteen-month-old child engaged in playing "gone–here." At certain times of the day, Freud relates, the child, who was not at all precocious, but well adjusted, flung into the corner of the room or under the bed all the small objects he could lay his hands on. With a gratified expression, he emitted a long drawn-out "o-o-o-o," which according to his mother meant "gone" (German, *"fort"*). The child was playing at being gone.

Some days later, Freud observed the same little boy playing with a reel tied to a piece of string. The game consisted in throwing the reel away from him, accompanying the action with an "o-o-o-o," and then in drawing it back, greeting its reappearance with a joyful "here" (German, *"da"*). It was, says Freud, a complete game centering around presence and absence, a fact which was confirmed on another day when the child greeted the return of his mother by "Baby o-o-o-o." Freud grasped the full meaning of the experience when he observed that during his long, solitary hours the child had invented another game; he had discovered his reflection in the mirror and was playing at *making himself disappear*.

Having first played at making his mother disappear, the child later played at losing himself. There are two phases involved here as far as identity is concerned. On the one hand, the child, very attached to the mother, seemed to await her return so that he could live anew independently of her; on the other hand, everything indicated from the outset that the child was sufficiently autonomous not to be disoriented by his mother's departure. He conjured up a word, probably his mother's, as she announced her departure: the game was punctuated by "gone" (*"fort"*) and "here" (*"da"*). It was probably in relation to his mother's words that the child was attempting to situate himself. The real mother disappeared and he put to the test the magic power of the word (the mother disappeared but the word remained). He could subsequently play at making himself disappear, because he was sure that his mother would return. The first knowledge that any child has of his mother is that she appears at his call and then disappears. It is always against a background of "not being there" that the mother desired by the child emerges. It was this dimension the child was apparently trying to reproduce in his game. When he played at disappearing himself, he was a real image to himself, but the word continued to be present. What was apparent from the "gone–here" game was that the Symbolic dimension had entered into the mother-child relationship. It is owing to the existence of this dimension that mastery can be acquired, the child acting-out on himself the abandonment and rejection in a context of childish omnipotence; it is he who is abandoned and who rejects, retaining within himself a sufficiently secure mother figure so as not to have to die at her departure in reality.

From 1908 to 1920, Freud treated play as poetic creation, and then he discovered the part played by the repetition principle, as a function of mastering unpleasant situations. He regarded play as a text to be decoded, even indicating the place the onlooker occupied in it. He had an inkling that it was an activity invested with emotion by the child, which could also arouse the feelings of the adult if it reached a certain standard as an esthetic creation. We find in his remarks all the conditions for observing the child closely, indeed for using this observation in treatment. Play became a "serious" form of expression because it was punctuated by a modulation of a voice, or a word.

The American school has taken up Freud's insights under the label of *play therapy,* but in some ways the significance of Freud's contribution has been missed. For Anna Freud, who did not work with the child's unconscious, but with his ego, analysis does not admit of fantasy as expression. Margaret Lowenfeld rejected any analytic dimension, her orientation being psychophysiological.[21] She saw only motor patterns in the child's play. In the United States, non-directive play therapy flourished. Children were invited to play, destroy, and wreck without a positive interpretation being attached to anything they did. They came to the therapy "to abreact their emotions."

After believing that this method would prove capable of curing the most deep-rooted disorders, some Americans reconsidered their position and admitted that "non-directive play therapy, though promising when evaluated subjectively, is seen as having rather serious methodological gaps." [22] With Erikson,[23] there was a return to Freud; the child gives evidence in his play of his psychological stance in a dangerous situation (this is equivalent to his defense mechanisms); the child expresses in play his setbacks, his unhappiness, and his frustrations, but this supposes a *language* of play, a language Erikson compares to cultural dialects or slang. He says the analyst must contrive to translate this language. However, we find two conceptions in Erikson's perceptive analysis which do not always coexist happily. If play is a language for him, he also gives equal stress to "behavior configurations," his observations then being classified as "morpho-analytic descriptions." Erikson, in the course of making common-sense observations, endeavors to point out the path for the therapist to follow if he wishes to achieve an understanding of the situation. Play is seen as a text to be deciphered at times by means of linguistic laws, and at other times as a sociocultural fact where we are dealing with the situation of a child at a given moment of his life under certain clearly defined cultural conditions. These two approaches are not necessarily mutually exclusive, provided that they are rigorously related to a structure of language. This Erikson does not do. He is torn among various

21 Adolf G. Woltmann, "Varieties of Play Techniques" in Mary R. Haworth, ed., *Child Psychotherapy* (New York, Basic Books, 1964).

22 Dell Lebo, in Haworth, *Child Psychotherapy,* p. 430.

23 Woltmann, "Varieties of Play Techniques."

philosophical influences, and he is open, on the level of theory, to the charge of having failed to make a clear-cut choice.

It is known that Melanie Klein introduced play into child analysis as early as 1919 while continuing to respect the rigorous nature of adult analysis in conducting treatment. She made use of a large number of small toys, and attached a certain importance to the child's choice. The interpretation she made, according to some writers, is an interpretation of *symbols*. If it were, it would certainly be the weakest point in Kleinian theory. Distorted in this manner, her writings would seem like a caricature of analysis, but it would betray her thought to read her in that way.

Let us return to Freud's observations in 1920. The child, as we saw, punctuated with a word what could be interpreted as the rejection and return of the mother. The words "gone" and "here" introduced a third dimension—beyond the absence of the real mother, the child found the Symbolic mother by means of a word. Then, with his body, the child began to try out the game of his own disappearance and return, that is, to lay down in relation to his mother's body and his own the bases of his identity. But the field in which he moved was a field of language in which his mother's words were disseminated. The object utilized by the child was a matter of indifference; he threw away all small objects within his reach, or used a reel. These substitute objects are not symbols but signifiers—they can be anything at all in themselves (they are not representational). It is only the use which the child made of them that throws light on his relationship with his mother—the experience he had not only of her presence and absence, but also of what was lacking in the relationship (the phallus). The child had absolutely no need, therefore, of a nursery full of toys. *He could contrive to convey his meaning with anything at all.*

The text he offered was a language; in that syntax functioned the overdetermination mechanisms whose effects, as they operate at the level of the text,[24] must be understood. We see the child, to be sure,

___

[24] J. Lacan, "Situation de la psychanalyse en 1956," in *Écrits* (Paris, Éditions du Seuil, 1966), p. 459.

with his gestures, motility, and an attitude full of meaning. But the attention of the analyst should be concentrated on discourse which is only partly verbal.

Let us reiterate. To decipher the text, we must integrate into it our resistance and that which serves in the child to screen his words, but we must also realize who is speaking, because the subject of the words is not necessarily the child. It is by following this line that we rediscover the meaning of the Freudian message—a message repeatedly forgotten and always to be rediscovered.

PART 1

PART 1

CHAPTER I

THE SYMPTOM OR THE WORD

The American school, under the influence of behaviorism, has emphasized the effect of conflicts between the subject and his surroundings. Are we to understand the neurotic symptom as the result of such interplay? And does that interpretation take us to the heart of what is really at issue in psychoanalysis?

Freud demonstrated the importance of the early years of life. The child must pass through necessary conflicts, which are identification conflicts, not conflicts with the *Real;* and if the external world is experienced by the child as benevolent or hostile in turn, we know that it is not a biological or animal situation, "a struggle for survival," but an *Imaginary* one which must be gradually *symbolized.*[1] In his relationship with his parents, the child has to learn to abandon a dual situation (which has Imaginary fascination) in

---

[1] *Symbolic:* Jacques Lacan distinguishes the *Symbolic* from the *Imaginary* and the *Real.* The Imaginary relationship with the other occurs in a dual situation which is primarily narcissistic. Aggressiveness and identification with the image of the other predominate at this stage. The *Symbolic* element is one that intervenes to break up an Imaginary relationship from which there is no way out. The child meets the "third element" upon birth; he enters a world ordered by a culture, law, and language, and is enveloped in that Symbolic order. (The meaning of *Symbolic* here is quite different from that of Jung's.) Finally, Lacan distinguishes the *Other,* the locus from which the code emanates, from the Imaginary *other.*

order to enter a ternary order—that is, to structure the Oedipus complex—which can come about only by his entry into the order of language.

Freud's contribution is to make us aware from the very first that in psychoanalysis it is not the case of an individual confronting the Real, nor is it his behavior; what is the case is the Imaginary failure of the self to recognize successive forms of identifications, snares, and alienations which represent the individual's defense against the approach of truth.

Child psychoanalysis does not differ in spirit (in listening) from the psychoanalysis of adults; but the adult, even the psychoanalyst himself, is often handicapped when he tackles the problems of childhood by his conception (Imaginary projection) of the problems. (Freud himself is not blameless in this respect.) All studies of childhood involve adults with all their reactions and prejudices.

The observations carried out by Françoise Dolto[2] of normal twenty-months-old infants suffering acute emotional tension at the birth of a sibling show the extent to which the adult is an active participant in the conflict. The child who is confused by the sudden loss of all his identity recognition points requires the right word, the "master word,"[3] to invoke in a state of crisis, so that he can establish control through it. The child demands the right to understand the things happening to him in one or another of his aggressive reactions which make no sense. The adult rarely observes this; he blames an *intention* whereas the child offers a form of behavior to be deciphered. Unable to make out its meaning, the adult leaves the child stifled with a desire for knowledge of the word, camouflaged by his claims or acts of rebellion. In two cases recounted by Françoise Dolto, it was possible for the child, in response to getting the right word, to present his own truth (murder fantasy) even in

---

[2] F. Dolto, "Hypothèses nouvelles concernant les réactions de jalousie à la naissance d'un puîné," *Psyché,* Nos. 7, 9, 10 (1947).

[3] The phrase used by a five-year-old child, as reported by F. Dolto.

the course of an attack of stammering; through the word, he emerged victorious from the conflict. (In a week's time, advances were observed in the field of language—he started to use tenses of verbs, his vocabulary was enriched, etc.)

In the case of Jean, Dolto relates a child's reactions during the three-week period following the birth of a brother. She describes the confusion expressed by bedwetting, soiling, and stammering. As the child continued to express his hostility and jealousy, the symptoms gradually disappeared. The stammering stopped on the twenty-first day when the child put a celluloid doll he called Guicha (his brother's name) in the maid's bed. He had slaughtered the doll in his mother's presence, thereby making her an accomplice in the symbolic murder of the brother who had arrived to take his place. As soon as he had done this, the child began to behave gently towards the object he had attacked, and subsequently to the baby. Although the stammering disappeared, Dolto notes that it is not easy to understand the mechanism brought into play in such attacks of defiance and aggressiveness. The symptom was presented as a message in code, and the mother was sufficiently understanding to allow herself to be marked by it. The "true word" expressing itself in the guise of the symptom was a murder fantasy, but not a murderous intention. The mother's intervention enabled the child to discard his "symptomatic" disguise and reveal the reverse side of the "true word": it was *also* an expression of love.

In the case of Gricha, we see a child confused in exactly the same way by the birth of a sister. He reacted by defiance, refusal to eat, bedwetting, and stammering. On the twenty-first day, he lay down in the baby's bed and acting, according to the mother, as if he were retarded, said, inanely, *"ma to tati"* ("me like Katy"). He wanted to keep his mother close. Dolto explains that here, again, it was by a sort of ritual murder that the child emerged victorious from his stammering—and his conflict. Both cases cast light on the identification conflict the child is exposed to. Any intervention by the adult to bring him back to normal serves only to lock the child into the regressive behavior which he chose for the purpose of staying the way he thinks his mother desires him.

In a similar case, a child became neurotic through the same type of experience, but Françoise Dolto notes that the misunderstanding arose on the language level; the adult was more anxious to correct jealous behavior than to reply to the child's questions. The child felt himself blamed for intentions he was assumed to have, and since he lost sight of his identity recognition points he fell prey to an inward disorder which he perceived as threatening.

In a persecutory situation, the child—a two-year-old boy named Robert—became dangerous for others. In three days, by sole virtue of the right words uttered by his mother, who was not neurotic, the child emerged cured from the attack, and at the same time acquired control in the field of language. It was in response to his mother's words that Robert had become dangerous to the baby. The interview with the analyst helped the mother to understand the tension behind his aggressive actions, which were dangerous yet devoid of murderous *intention,* and she was then able to modify her choice of words with the child. She put into *words* the aggressiveness of the boy but without condemning it, as if she herself were assuming responsibility for it. Upon his recovery Robert started to side with his baby brother, and reproached his mother for her wickedness. The mother's *words* made it possible for him to situate himself whereas in the earlier phase, unable to cope with the tension engulfing him, the child had been destroying himself.

The interest of these observations lies in the fact that they reveal the child in a crisis situation as it is unfolding, and the adult in a situation of responding to it according to his own fantasies, prejudices, or educational principles. In the case of Robert who became "difficult," the mother wanting to shut her eyes to his jealousy was unable to find the right words. She had done everything, in effect, to prevent the child from becoming jealous, thus moving the pawns into position according to her desire; the child, in introducing his own desire, overturned the board, especially since he had been forbidden to play that particular game of chess. "Mummy knows what is good for him." The right word is not easy to bring out; it refers the mother back to her own recognition points. If replies are going to be foreclosed, the child will find it difficult to put his question, except in the form of behavior disorders.

I should like to try to cast some light on this problem, by way of Freud's famous study of "Little Hans." [4] What interests me is not the analysis of the case but the fragments of observation by the father which highlight the screens the adult erects so as to keep the child in a state of *unknowing*. The observation begins with a question Hans addresses to his mother, "Mummy, have you got a widdler *too?*" The ambiguous term—designating as it does both the urinary and sexual functions of the organ—was one employed by the mother. She took good care not to use another that might designate both her sexual organ and the one she lacked. Still, all of Hans's questions during the first part of the observation bore palpably on what the mother *had* or *did not have*. The child hunted for the appropriate word, despite countless rebuffs. He was prepared to say something wrong so as to have the *true* word revealed (or restored) to him. In actuality, Hans, at the age of three, *knew* the essential difference between the sexes, yet he did not dare to allow himself the right to this knowledge which was foreclosed by the adult's wish. Consequently, when the mother replied with a half-truth—"Of course. Why?"—the child had no words to translate what he thought. "I was just thinking," he said to the adult who was not listening to him.

We see from that observation how Hans, who had not yet become neurotic, mystified *himself* every time he came up against adult resistance. To keep his self-respect, which was derived from the Other, he reframed his question, or rather his answer, on the level at which the adult was willing to accept it. He bestowed on

[4] S. Freud, "Analysis of a Phobia in a Five-Year-Old Boy," in Standard Edition, Vol. X. My reflections on "Little Hans" have been inspired by an original work by F. Dolto, presented to a study group at L'École freudienne in May, 1965.

himself the mystifying word that responded appropriately to the adult's desire.

Let us work through the situation again. Occasionally, Hans's quest for the right word had a tinge of anxiety; it subsumed at the time of his baby sister's birth Hans's whole position in the face of his parents' desire. He was clearly looking for recognition points,[5] but his task was made very difficult because his father referred him to his mother for points of reference, implying thereby that when it came to sex, the question was to be posed in terms of the mother's ideal. As it happens, the mother liked little girls, although she regarded her son's genitals as "a pretty little machine," and she talked about it to her best friend. Hans's sexual parts were an object to be looked at for the adult, but which he himself could not touch; they were something of concern to others, or rather to be tolerated as the functional urinary organ but condemned as Hans's seat of desire. Now, the question underlying Hans's incursions into the field of language was, What is desirable? The mother's response to the erotic situation that she herself had created by her attentions to the child was that he mustn't touch it, "That's dirty." This implies that she was concerned about Hans's sexual parts only in order to devalue them on the narcissistic level. She wanted her son's genitals to be a urinary organ, and not the seat of desire. Hans tried vainly to get his father to disavow his mother's words, and to put an ethical value on desire. His father condemned Hans to remain confronted by the meaninglessness of being merely a passive object loved by a mother who does not desire a man. She herself took part in play involving body contact with her son while she verbally condemned everything connected with sex. In effect, the mother's desire was that Hans should not be master of his masculine desire.

Freud relates that Hans's disorder, a dread of horses, appeared at the age of four years and nine months. It began with the fear that his mother would go away. "I thought you were gone and I had no Mummy to fondle me." This sudden anxiety was probably super-

---

[5] After the birth of a younger sibling, the child does not know whether he can continue to grow or whether he should stay little to conform with the adults' desire.

imposed on discussions between the parents which Hans had perhaps *heard*. The importance he attached to the words that he might
have overheard was all the greater because in reality he was being
frustrated by his mother's silence. The mother did not tell him that
she had no desire for her husband; she disguised the truth—the
danger of her leaving—by clinging to her son, to the idea of the
nice little boy. As soon as Hans left his mother, anxiety prevailed.
His genitals, the locus of tension, belonged to his mother, to be
looked at by her. The child was arrested in his masculine evolution; he was walled in by his mother's desire of not desiring a man,
and by his father's desire of seeing him conform to his mother's
wishes. Both parents were voyeurs of their child's genitals and of
his desire. They joked about his desire, it formed the subject of
conversation between adults, it was the link between the father and
Freud. The father did not talk to Freud about his own
sexuality—he talked about his son's, which is to say, his own,
lived through the sex of his child. By the same token, it was
through Hans that the mother tackled her problems with her best
friend.

"Is it all right or not to like playing with little girls?" was the
veiled question Hans addressed to his father. The father confined
himself to noting, for the sake of Freud, the birth of desire in his
son; he recognized Hans's difficulty but left him perplexed. Sex
remained an enigma.

The child gave his mother to understand that he knew the difference between the urinary and sexual functions of the penis, but he
found himself blocked by a position of refusal; the mother appeared to be saying, "If that is the case, I no longer love you," and
the child to be replying, "That's too bad." [6] Hans lacked the support

[6] Hans: "Well, then I'll just go downstairs and sleep with Mariedl."
Mother: "You really want to go away from Mummy and sleep downstairs?"
Hans: "Oh, I'll come up again in the morning to have breakfast and go to the
toilet."
Mother: "Well, if you really want to go away from Daddy and Mummy, then
take your coat and knickers and good-bye!"
Hans did take his clothes and go towards the staircase, to go and sleep with
Mariedl but, it need hardly be said, he was fetched back.

of his father and thus did not feel entitled to get out of the dual situation in which the mother wanted to imprison him.

The arrival of a new maid enabled Hans to regain his confidence in his own body just as he was giving in to the regressive proposal of his father that he sleep in a sleeping bag to suppress all temptation of desire. He was able to talk to the maid about her nudity, because she accepted the fact that she was a being without a penis, without running the risk of being threatened with mutilation, as was the case with his mother—"If you do that I shall send for Dr. A. to cut off your widdler." Hans could now show his power. The maid was content to be the locus of lack, and from that fact Hans gained the possibility of reinforcement on the narcissistic level. Thus when his father said to him, "You were probably frightened when you once saw the horse's big widdler. But there's no need for you to be frightened of it; big animals have big widdlers, and little animals have little widdlers," Hans could now reply, "Everyone has a widdler. And my widdler will get bigger as I get bigger; it's fixed in, of course." From then on, an adult could threaten him with castration, but he knew that *desire* itself continues to exist. For it was in fact desire that the child had introduced, confronted by a father who confined himself to observing the size of widdlers of large and small animals, and who subsequently did not dare to explain to his son the part played by the father in procreation.

Hans: "But I belong to you."

Father: "But Mummy brought you into the world, so you belong to Mummy and me."

Hans: "Does Anna belong to me or to Mummy?"

Father: "To Mummy."

Hans: "No, to me. Why not to Mummy and me?"

Father: "Anna belongs to me, Mummy, and you."

Hans: "So there!"

Let us explore this a little further. In actuality, Hans suspected from the outset the genital implications of the two sexes, but his father refused to reveal them to him. Hans was not given the words he was entitled to expect. There was unwillingness to tell him that he was born of a father and a mother, yet he needed this truth so that a masculine identification could assume meaning. Hans acquired for himself the answer which the adult refused him, by using a fantasy theme as a go-between: "When there's one horse and the cart's loaded full up, then I'm afraid; but when there are two horses and it's loaded full up, then I'm not afraid." He signified thereby that he *knew* that procreation is not the act of the mother on her own. In this rich observation the following point should be stressed: It was at the time—towards the age of three— when Hans was becoming aware of his body in being proud of his male sexual organ that the mother intervened to rob him of his narcissism. She reduced the sense of the sexual organ to something purely functional; it was an organ to make pipi with, it was a dirty thing, and all that had nothing to do with fertility. This happened at a time when Hans needed to feel that he was born of the union of a father and a mother, in order to become aware of himself as a boy.

What he was trying to discern in both parents was their position towards desire, so that he could orient himself according to a scale of values. But the only scale of values suggested to him was the passive maternal ideal of being a nice cuddly little boy. The thirst for knowledge in Hans was directly linked to his investigations of sex, which is to say, of the meaning of his existence: Where did I come from? What should I aim at? It was the child's own resources that made up for the deficiency caused by the inadequacy of adult response by a succession of mythical themes. He succeeded, at the cost of a phobia, in imposing his knowledge on the adult or, if he could not, then in mystifying *himself* rather than being mystified. This implied, at any rate, a form of inward liberation and safeguarded his intellectual potentialities. "I'm lying to myself," the child seemed to be saying, "so I can go on asking myself questions beyond the lie as long as I respect a rule of the game, which is, to behave *as if* I didn't understand a thing." Freud's intervention, putting the father's desire into words ("Even before you were born, I knew that your father wanted a son"), was certainly decisive in bringing the child the help he had been seeking in vain from an adult. By introducing in this way the wish from the father's pre-existence Freud made it possible for Hans to recognize his debt to his father. The child's speech was on the level that adults could tolerate from him, and Hans periodically countered their deception with deception of his own. It was because the child was at the point of almost conscious self-deception that he preserved his intelligence, even though at the cost of a neurotic episode; deprived of the right to express himself truthfully in language, he revealed what he had to say by his symptom. The symptom became a secret language to which he kept the key. It is not the myths about storks or cabbages that trouble children but the deception of adults who put on an air of *speaking truthfully* and thus block the child from following up his intellectual incursions.

Hans's parents, who were having difficulties with their own sex life, wanted to regain in him the myth of a "pure" or "perverse" childhood—the expression of adult repression or projections. Actually, Hans was neither the ingenuous infant who wanted "to be left alone with his pretty mummy" nor the perverted one constantly in quest of various forms of sexual titillation. That creature emanated from the fantasy world of the father and mother. The child wanted a father to rely on. He was afraid, on the other hand, that his mother would abandon him, and he was prepared to develop a phobia to express his anxiety which was at the same time a fear of being imprisoned in a dual situation from which there was no out-let. Hans instinctively knew what he needed in order to live; he expressed it as far as he could in words and, when they failed, in his symptom.

The history of "Little Hans" is that of a child confronting an adult myth. It was the *word* of the adult that marked him and determined subsequent changes in his personality. The child served as the prop of adult fantasies and voyeurism. He was growing up in a world where the *unspoken* conveyed an awkward situation, a parental drama that the child was distinctly aware of. The traumatizing factor in a neurosis, as far as it can be pinned down, is never a *real* event in itself but what was said or left unsaid about it by the people concerned. It is the words, or absence of them, with which the painful scene is associated that provide the subject with the elements that strike his imagination. In the case of the "Wolf Man," [7] the mother's exclamation, "I cannot go on living like this," was associated with stomach disorders in which blood played a role, and which the child witnessed. "The mother's sufferings," says Freud, "made a deep impression on him, and later on he applied them to himself." In fact, we later see the subject suffering from the hallucination of losing a finger and having, as an adult, delusional preoccupations about his nose, which formed a veritable body of fantasy and made him repeat the words of his mother: "I cannot go on living like this."

A psychoanalytic cure is not unlike the unfolding of a mythical story. It is possible to recover in the subject's past the words of the mother linked to a physical reaction in the child which locate the trauma, and remain as a mark imprinted in the subject's speech. The fantasy, indeed the symptom itself, appears as a mask which serves to conceal the original text or the disturbing event. So long as the subject remains alienated in his fantasy, the disorder is revealed on the Imaginary level. In the case of Hans, it was his phobia of horses, and in the case of the Wolf Man, it was his phobias leading finally to his alienation in a fantasied body. The symptom, as Freud shows, always includes the subject *and* the Other. It is a situation in which the patient tries to indicate by means of a castration fantasy how he locates himself in relation to the desire of the Other. "What does he want me to do?" is the question behind all somatic disorders. The doctor's task is to bring out the questions the subject is unknowingly posing, but in order to do it he must be capable of "listening" elsewhere than at the actual site of the attack.

[7] S. Freud, "History of an Infantile Neurosis," in Standard Edition, Vol. XVII.

Erikson[8] gives a remarkable example of this in a study of a crisis, originally diagnosed as neurological, in a five-year-old child named Sam. Erikson's purpose is to demonstrate that a disturbing psychological event may lie at the root of a symptom which appears to be organic. It would seem that the interconnection of psychological and somatic factors constitutes a problem in itself which must not be overlooked. The originality of Erikson's approach, however, lies in his endeavor to get the "illness" to "speak." He regards it as a situation involving both the subject and the people around him. In order to understand the dynamics, Erikson sought to penetrate the patient's fantasy world. He states that if the analyst remains on the outside, he can in effect give but a description of the phenomenon, which has no therapeutic value. When one has located the cause of pathology, one cannot simply wash one's hands of the patient and his "illness." Treatment has no meaning, Erikson shows, unless we can plumb the problem (the theme of death in the present case), not only in the child but also in the parents. Consequently, we do not reconstruct a real past, but follow the development of a mythical theme in which the patient and his family, all unknowingly, have their place. It is of little importance that Erikson's interpretation of his analysis of the case reflects ethnographical and educational tendencies. His conduct of the treatment is so rigorous that he can pinpoint material which will place the situation in sharp focus. Throughout the presentation of the case, we are aware of the various permutations of the original theme—even when the author does not stress them. Articulated and re-articulated, these permutations enable us to understand in exactly what terms the child and his mother confront the unconscious question, "What does he want me to do?"—and to see how the fantasies of one need the support of the Other in order to evolve.

When Erikson entered the fantasy link between mother and child, their verbal interaction shifted in the direction of the analyst,

[8] Erikson, *Childhood and Society.*

making sense of what had been aggressive behavior or somatic manifestation. From the outset of treatment, Erikson's clinical instinct led him to concentrate on the motive of death; he correctly discerned it as the factor that triggered Sam's crisis, as the child's first attack had in fact begun five days after his grandmother's death. He followed the path as it led both in the child and his mother, from real facts to fantasy worlds in which, one might say, the word has a deadly effect, were it not more accurate to describe it as revealing the unconscious wish. We should note that we are given only a fragment of the analysis. Our information is limited to certain stages in the treatment, because Erikson is careful to present only such parts of clinical cases as serve to illustrate the actual objective of his book, the study of childhood and of social patterns in various ethnic groups. What impresses me particularly is the precision of his analytic approach, and I will attempt to summarize the points that are, in my opinion, the essential ones in the case.

1. Sam was three years old when his mother found him gripped in a posture that resembled that of the heart attack his grandmother had died of five days earlier. The doctor diagnosed epilepsy, sent him to a hospital for observation, and he stayed there a few days. His neurological reflexes were normal, and there was apparently nothing to report.

2. *One month later,* the boy found a dead mole. That night he vomited repeatedly and displayed symptoms of an epileptic episode. The hospital to which he was sent hypothesized a cerebral lesion in the left hemisphere.

3. *Two months later,* a third attack occurred after the boy had crushed a butterfly in his hand. The hospital amended its previous tentative diagnosis and suggested that the precipitating factor might have been a psychic stimulus. The doctor was struck by the common factor in the three episodes; namely the connection between the deaths of the grandmother, the mole, and the butterfly, and the ensuing epileptic attacks. Since no organic cause could be detected (the electroencephalogram merely indicated that epilepsy

"could not be excluded"), Erikson applied himself to apprehending the part played by the idea of death in the child's life. First, he set out to determine the facts surrounding the grandmother's death and questioned the mother about it.

He learned that the young woman had been feeling overwrought at that time. The recent arrival of her mother-in-law had been worrying her, because she was concerned about being criticized by the older woman. Also, she was troubled by Sam's unruliness in view of her mother-in-law's heart condition. Sam liked to tease, and she was afraid he would tire the old lady.

It was while the mother was absent that the grandmother was stricken, and after reconstructing the facts it seemed likely that the child had been tiresome and teasing during her absence. In an interview the mother recalled that the night before his "attack" Sam had carefully piled up his pillows as he had seen his grandmother do for herself. She insisted, however, that Sam was not supposed to know anything about his grandmother's death. He was told that she had gone on a long journey, and Sam cried and said, "Why didn't she say good-bye to me?" The purpose of the coffin had to be accounted for, also, and Sam was told that it was a box for his grandmother's books. Erikson doubted that the boy really believed his mother's explanations, and he conveyed his skepticism to her. She then remembered an incident which occurred during that time; she had asked the boy to find something that he did not want to look for, and he said mockingly, "It has gone on a long, long trip to Seattle." Later on, he refused categorically to listen to any of his mother's explanations about his grandmother's death. "That's not true, you're lying," he said. "She's in Seattle. I'm going to find her again."

During subsequent interviews the mother remembered a detail she had forgotten to mention: Sam had been forced to keep his grandmother company by way of punishment, with a warning against teasing her. The boy had hit a playmate, a little blood had trickled, and it seemed like a good idea to keep Sam at home to prevent trouble outside.

What interested Erikson in this account was the "aggressive" characteristics of the Jewish ethnic minority group to which Sam's family belonged. They had broken with their ancestral tradition and had moved to a Gentile neighborhood where they were trying to outdo their neighbors in "respectability." The family seemed to have brought its influence to bear on the child to restrain his over-impulsiveness and to behave "nicely" like the Gentile children.

Erikson began treating Sam two years after the onset of the illness, and he noted the following stages:

1. During an analytic session the boy became furious at having lost a game of dominoes and threw something at Erikson's face. Then he grew very pale, and seemed about to vomit. Pulling himself together, he said, "Let's go on." By means of a transference process Erikson gave him the interpretation of his upset:

a. "If you wanted to see the dots on your dominoes in the box you've built with them, you'd have to be inside the box like a dead person in a coffin."

b. The child having answered "yes," Erikson went on, "Perhaps you're afraid that you may have to die because you hit me."

c. "Must I?" asked Sam, and Erikson replied, "Of course not." He went on to point out the parallel between the grandmother's death and Sam's fear that he had made her die. The child accepted it. He had never before admitted that he knew his grandmother was dead. Here, Erikson remarks, we have the precipitating cause of the illness, but we cannot stop at this point.

2. Erikson undertook to work with the mother; he maintains that the psychic origin of disorder in a young child invariably has its corollary in a neurotic conflict in the mother. He places this specific neurotic conflict in a sociocultural context involving the family's break with Jewish tradition, the mother's feelings of guilt towards her father, and the unreasonable demand on the boy to be like non-Jews. Sam threw a doll at his mother's face and broke a tooth. She hit him in a rage such as she had never displayed before. Erikson points out that she had exacted "a tooth for a tooth," as it were, although on the plane of reality she had not.

At this point, Erikson asked to have a talk with both parents together. The interview bears on the history of the couple and covers their past money troubles, present worries, and future ambitions.

3. A few days later, Sam climbed on his mother's knees and said, "Only a very bad boy would want to jump on his mommy and step on her. . . . Only a very bad boy would want to do that, isn't that so, Mommy?" The mother reacted by laughing and said, "I bet you would like to do it right now. I think a very good little boy might think he wanted to do such a thing, but he would know he did not really want to do it." "Yes," answered the boy, "I won't do it. There won't be any scene tonight, Mommy."

It was in the same way that Little Hans said that wanting to do is not the same as doing; in this case, the mother undramatized for her son everything that related to his unconscious death-wish.

What can we now extricate from this rich material? Erikson presents a *method* of investigation and of conducting treatment. He is not concerned in this book with technical problems as they might pose themselves to the analyst. His examples, let me repeat, serve to illustrate his study on the social significance of childhood. Yet, it is as an analyst that I was responsive to the clinical presentation of the case. Let us follow it. The *real fact*—the trauma produced by the grandmother's death—has no importance for Erikson on the level of pure research into the cause of the "illness." It must be made to assume a meaning. The clinical process consists of two phases (here Erikson follows Freud): the period of investigation and the treatment proper.

During the investigatory period Erikson isolates the principal themes to be taken up in treatment. In Sam's case, it was through the theme of death that the mother expressed her guilt (the fear of being criticized) and her shame (the fear that her son would not grow up to be like a non-Jew). The death itself, occurring after Sam's teasing, made her so uneasy that she was induced to deny the event, and consequently she burdened her son with being accessory to a lie. She made a deceptive remark to Sam in order to justify her part in the incident, and then recalled that it had failed to dupe Sam. As for Sam, he answered deception with deception while appearing to know very well what it was all about.

In the course of treatment, the mother brought in the recollection of the rage aroused by her son's mutilation of her, by breaking a tooth. There was between them a settling of accounts, as it were, and this incident referred the mother back to her own unconscious death-wishes and to the castration problem. An interview with both parents enabled Erikson to perceive the conflict this Jewish couple had been engulfed by. They were both caught between forebears they had more or less disowned on the one hand, and on the other, a child whom they expected not to identify himself with his Jewish lineage. They wanted Sam to be a nice boy and non-Jewish, but the child showed himself to be impulsive and pugnacious instead, not good "like other people's children." Erikson presents only a few details of the interview with the parents; yet it seems to have been a turning point, for it was from this juncture—the day the father entered into the child's treatment—that the mother could say the true words relating to *desire:* "Thinking you want to do something isn't the same as doing it." Sam was receptive to these words, which gave him the right to have guilty thoughts and at the same time granted him a sort of autonomy. He could now have a desire without his mother. In terms of the transference situation, he received a response bearing on his identification with the grandmother and at the same time offering proof of his fear that his aggressiveness was lethal.

Sam's difficulties unfolded on two levels. In the first place, he *was* his mother's symptom in the sense that she felt herself judged through him, and if she deceived him, as she had, it was because she herself wished to deny the grandmother's death. In the second place, Sam was the subject within his symptom: "What am I to be to please my mother?" His mother required him in effect to disown his ancestry, which made it difficult for him to identify with a

39

masculine image. She was asking him not to be like his father, but like a dream child, the "good child" of non-Jewish mothers.

The grandmother's death assumed importance to the extent that the mother felt herself designated as the murderer through her son. There was no longer any other solution for the boy but to become victim so as not to be executioner.

This part of the analysis was not carried far enough to enable us to get more out of it. We find in it the same themes I have attempted to highlight in the analysis of Little Hans: The important factor is not the real event but the deception by the adult concerning it. The child finds himself faced with the dilemma of either denouncing the deception, which will save him, or mystifying himself to the extent required to support a mystification needed by the adult.[9]

Erikson's approach is different from that of Freud. In Little Hans's case, the father, through the person of Freud, appointed himself his child's analyst in a relationship in which he was nevertheless the unconscious voyeur of his son's disorders, in order to report the facts back to Freud, on whom he had a fixation. The mother probably felt herself excluded from a dialogue, and she carried on a sort of constant deception with her son which cancelled out the work done elsewhere.

Erikson gave a hearing to both parents, and in particular to the mother; therefore, she no longer needed her son to express her own problem—the break with her ancestry. The work with the child was an example of a classical analysis, but Erikson does not tell us if he pursued it to its conclusion. The importance he attaches to sociocultural factors leads him perhaps to lose sight of the strictly analytical meaning that such factors can assume in treatment, and which justify their being explored. The important aspect of Sam's case is not so much the history of an uprooted Jewish couple as the part played by the child in his parents' fantasies. It was the parents' wish to break with their Jewish ancestry that produced an identifi-

9 *See* O. Mannoni, "Je sais bien . . . mais quand même," *Les Temps modernes,* No. 212 (January, 1964).

cation problem in Sam. Therefore, it was not astonishing that some progress was achieved in treatment as soon as the Name of the Father and the idea of death were introduced, a fact Erikson passes over in his theoretical conclusions. And yet, in his clinical material, we see that the analysis develops strictly along "traces," "signifiers," and "recognition points." [10] It is regrettable therefore that there is no link between the quality of the clinical work and the theory; Erikson displays the clinical material in the treatment, but he employs it only from the sociocultural viewpoint.

I think I have made it clear in my presentation of Sam's case that social factors play a smaller part than Erikson appears to believe. The problem is not the situation of a Jewish family in a Gentile environment, but the mother-child link in the mother's fantasy relationship. The child's situation in that particular role did not escape Erikson's notice as he was "listening" to the family as a clinician. He gave weight to the forgotten word, to what remained unsaid, he advanced relentlessly upon the themes that were important both for mother and for child; but, he leaves the clinic when he works out his theories, which never appear to be the natural extension of the text we have been reading. He dissects society and its traditions, although he knew how to "listen" in another quarter in his role as analyst. It would be instructive to make a closer study of the technical problems of conducting treatment through Erikson's clinical cases, but to do that one would have to have access to the details of the original text, namely, the patient's words. In extricating the essential points from such material Lacan's criteria have been more helpful to me than Erikson's sociological principles. Lacan's criteria help to impose order on the patient's words in cases where the themes threaten to become submerged under considerations too far removed from the clinic.

On the clinical level, Erikson is not handicapped by prejudices, which enables him to make discoveries. But when he attempts to go more deeply into what happens during treatment on another level, the conceptualization he relies on falls far short of its clinical

[10] Terms employed by Bernfeld, Lacan, and Melanie Klein, respectively.

potential. Erikson is speaking about experience and relationships when he stresses, quite rightly, the forgotten word. His theories, in which language is regarded as a communication, lead him to emphasize the study of interpersonal links, whereas what emerges on the level of observation is that which is unfolding in the patient's words. We have seen how Sam was changed by language in the course of treatment; what he said was first a denial and then an acceptance of death. It was in his language that he made plain his impossible position within his mother's dream. Gradually, and to the extent that the words ceased to be mystifying, Sam shifted his position in relation to the desire of the Other. He was no longer under the Imaginary influence of an unconscious death-wish—his own and his mother's. Although Erikson renders the patient's words, he does not undertake to study them at the textual level. It is *patterns,* habits, education, and customs that attract him. He is preoccupied with the problem of communication[11] and that is the fountainhead of his inquiries and researches.

Lacan, on the contrary, studies the manner in which the subject is changed by language—a conception that does not allow for a thought which is anterior to the word. In this he follows the pointers offered by Freud in the "Rat Man" and the "Wolf Man": fantasy consists of a word which is sometimes lost to consciousness under the fantastic effects conjured up by it. This thesis can be proved clinically, as I have attempted to show.

The problem of *communication* was referred to by Freud [12] in a remark pointing out the child's belief in the omnipotence of the thought of the adult, to whom he ascribes the power of reading his thoughts. In "Dreams and Occultism" [13] he quotes a story told by

[11] What is involved is the communication between the mother's thought and the child's; Freud went so far as to consider a hypothesis, which seems far-fetched to us, of a transmission along the same lines as telepathy. The origin of such beliefs lies evidently in the child's own illusion that the adult knows his thoughts (see the case of the "Rat Man").

[12] *See* footnote 11 above.

[13] S. Freud, "Dreams and Occultism" in Vol. XXII, Standard Edition.

an analyst who had been treating a mother and her child. On two separate occasions, the child brought his mother a gold coin just as the mother was verbalizing to the analyst about the important part played by a certain other gold coin during her own childhood. The first time, the child asked his mother to keep the coin for him. The second time, he wanted it back in order to *talk* about it during his own analytic session—at the very moment when his mother was ready to want to write down for the analyst an exact account of the facts, so as *to be able to talk about them.*

Freud recounts this story in concluding a series of similar stories collected by people interested in the occult sciences; he expresses no opinion based on them. These accounts seemed to him to raise the problem of *thought transmission.* If Freud was led, not without offering resistance, to a hypothesis of thought transmission, it was because he could not see how anything in the *overt* behavior of the mother could explain the communication of her fantasies to the child. Concerning the anecdote of the gold coin, Freud does not attach much importance to thought transmission; he tells us in plain language that the story refers us back to a problem of analysis, thus emphasizing that if an enigma does exist, the key to it will be found in the field of analysis. The little gold coin, an element *common to* mother and son to the extent of playing a part in a certain fantasy relationship, is then taken up again *so that it can be talked about*—to a third party, the analyst. Freud's passing remark therefore leads us to words, and his inquiries stop there. He could not say more about the case than had been related to him. English and American analysts have become interested in this problem, to which Freud had no answer. Everyone has experienced in his analytic work "coincidences" like those in the story of the gold coin. Might the child not have perceived [14] in the overt behavior of his mother an incoherent element, a special signal that dictated his re-

[14] Ilse Hellman *et al.,* "Simultaneous Analysis of a Mother and Child," in *The Psychoanalytic Study of the Child,* Vol. XV (New York, International Universities Press; London, Imago, 1960).

sponse (response to behavior which is out of place)? The parent's unconscious wish is thus to be read in actions, and not in *words*. This hypothesis would reduce one to supposing that certain manifestations which Freud (or the analyst) should have recognized have quite simply escaped him, or that they occurred outside his field of observation. If analysts reject, and rightly so, the thesis of thought transmission, they expose themselves to another danger in adopting a flatly positivist theory which holds that in fact there exists no communication between mother and child which we adults cannot recognize as overt. In this baffling form of communication, which in fact does exist, the child's unconscious is made aware of what the mother desires or refuses, to a certain point. We have seen in the analysis of Little Hans how the child reacted not so much to the adult's attitude as to her words and silences. The adult observer can only see what he calls the "overt" in the mother's remarks, but the child, less repressed, gets a richer message. To read the message, one must disentangle oneself from a reality which is always deceptive—in Hans's case, the father comparing the sizes of small and large widdlers—in order to shift the questioning over to desire—it was desire that Hans was trying to introduce when he tracked down the desire of the Other. This leads us to lay stress on the importance to be accorded in treatment to *fantasy,* which should be understood not as the image or trace of an experience lived through, but rather as a word lost.

In "Further Remarks on the Defence Neuro-Psychoses," [15] Freud cites the case of an eleven-year-old boy who had devised an obsessional ceremony at bedtime, which was directed at his mother. Among other things, he had to tell her the events of the day in the minutest detail. But, by these words, which he made as accurate as possible, he clung desperately to an entire context of realities that assumed importance only because it was *in place of* what he wanted to admit but dared not, namely, the maid's desire for him and the sexual seductions to which he had been subjected. The

[15] In Standard Edition, Vol. III.

observation is brief; we see the true word being transformed into what might be called symptomatic speech (detailed confession) which, although it is speech, does not differ from other symptoms. (The boy was driven to say how much he liked a clean floor, and he protected himself by a rampart of chairs and pillows intended to prevent someone from getting into his bed again, that is to say, the resumption of sex play.) The symptom took the place of the words that were lacking. The child introduced into the dialogue his position in relation to his mother's desire—a clean floor—because that particular desire was of no consequence; *that was not the point at issue.* What was at issue, neither one nor the other could or would touch on. The symptom occurred as a mask or a code word. The mother was party to the symptom. The important point in Freud's observation is that we see the *symptom accompanied by the deceptive words.* Why did the boy seek to "give" his mother false words? Were they the expression of her own wish? What link existed between the story of seduction (which the boy was so eager to relate) and an incestuous mother-son desire? The boy, like Little Hans, was *without words* to express what he thought. Instead of what he had to say he only produced the symptom, in this case more deceptive words or, more precisely, a riddle to be solved. The symptom was addressed to the mother, that is to say, it touched on her personal position in regard to a certain knowledge about sex. The child felt confusedly that he did not have the right to communicate to his mother a certain knowledge which she did not wish to hear. The mask, the symptom, was the use of a code language specially created for the person to whom it was addressed. Erikson understood this fact completely from the clinical viewpoint. He listened to what was being said through the symptom, but in giving his account he was blocked by current theories of development and its vicissitudes, which naturally lead on to the emphasis of environmental influence. We have seen above that the explanation he gives, though highly interesting, does not reflect what happened during treatment; it was not a matter of an ethnic conflict but the subject's

45

own question, put by means of the symptom from the locus of the Other.

"When he asks the question," says Lacan about the analysis of a text,[16] " 'What does that cough mean?' it is a question twice removed from the event. It is a question that arises from the Other, since it is to the extent that he is in analysis that he begins to ask it. It is a question literally concerning the other inside him, concerning his unconscious. 'What is this signifier of the Other within me?' "

By distinguishing the Real from the Imaginary and the Symbolic Lacan has made it possible to avoid misinterpretation in the clinical approach. In focusing treatment on the manner that the subject situates himself in relation to the Other's desire, Lacan makes it possible to grasp on the theoretical plane what is happening to, and what is alien to the subject's relationships with reality or with the people around him. This process is "the communication of the subject to the dimension of language as such, arising from the fact that he has to situate himself as subject in speech to make himself manifest as *being* through it." [17] Viewed in this perspective, the symptom does indeed seem to be a word through which the subject indicates in an enigmatic way how he situates himself in relation to all forms of desire. The concept of the symptom, as it is expressed in Lacan's work, challenges the classical nosology[18] which is based on the separation of the doctor and the patient, and on a therapeutics originating in the submission of a particular experience of the patient to the reliable judgment of the doctor.

What the doctor fails to grasp in this relationship is precisely the factor on which the subject relies to explain himself, thus making himself, in his symptom, a recognition signifier. Erikson's attainment is that, on the clinical level, he avoided being therapeutically ineffectual by listening to what was spoken precisely where it was

[16] J. Lacan, in seminar, January 21, 1959 (unpublished).

[17] J. Lacan, in seminar, June 17, 1959. A summary was published in the *Bulletin de psychologie,* Vol. XIII, Nos. 5–6 (January, 1960), "Le Désir et son interprétation."

[18] J. Lacan, in seminar, July 1, 1959 (unpublished).

actually "speaking"—in the symptom. However, since his conceptualization remained attached to a traditional theory, he could not
go closely into what was really happening from the subject's viewpoint. He believes that the patient is to be changed by his surroundings whereas we see him as being "remodeled" by language.

II [19]

If Erikson, owing to his intuition as clinician, was able to escape
from a narrowly medical attitude in which inquiries bear on facts
rather than on being, it is the fate of other theorists, not yet rescued
from certain philosophical tenets inherited from the nineteenth
century, to be prevented from a proper understanding of a case by
their ideas about theory. We see them asking questions of human
"reality" and of behavior, divided as they are between biological
determinism and culturalist theories. Explanations are given at
points where the "facts" ought not be described but queried, so as
to reveal the subject's question.

In a work on infantile psychosis[20] we see the extent to which
certain theoretical notions can handicap analysts in their "listening." Committed to a preconceived idea about a given situation
they record fully what is said, but the meaning eludes them. The
authors present us with what is virtually a shorthand record of the
sessions, but lacking a framework for arranging the material, the
essential themes get lost. The faithful record at the level of the Real
contrasts with the failure to record at the level of meaning. The
child's words are transcribed like a step in a factual experiment,
and they are objectified in order to be submitted subsequently for
the doctor's experienced judgment. The production of fantasy is
thus converted into a literary production[21] in which no analysis of
the words is undertaken.

[19] This section was published in *Revue de psychothérapie institutionnelle,* No. 4.

[20] S. Lebovici and J. McDougall, *Un Cas de psychose infantile* (Paris, Presses
Universitaires de France, 1960).

[21] The child was allowed to take home what he had dictated to the analyst. The
text thus became a document "given" to the adults so that they could discuss it
between themselves.

The analyst holds the discussion at the level of objects; the very words are petrified, fixed in their position like things. The subject need not form himself by his words, nor make himself accessible through them; he is asked to live in an experimental relationship, in order to become adjusted to a style of life recognized as normal. Instead of examining the actual words closely, thereby helping the child to cast up the signifier elements—here again, as it happens, the theme of death—speech becomes a sort of still life whose significance the analyst recognizes from his knowledge. In this way we get diagrams which explain the child's fixation at such and such a stage in his psychological development, a stage at which occur such and such "drives and defense mechanisms," such and such a "structure of the ego," or "psychotic object relationship"; in this perspective, drawings, too, take on a "meaning," which is explained.[22]

This technique is founded on a psychoanalytic theory related to psychophysical parallelism. The analyst, as observer, stays outside the patient's field, as the latter becomes objectified in his words and behavior. In his role as patient, he is subject to the adult's sane judgment. He is a subject-object, called upon to "get well" if he becomes aware of what is pathogenic in his conduct. He is urged to rehabilitate himself. The analytic criteria are based on a belief in a strong or weak ego, called on to oppose more or less powerful instinctual forces. All such ideas mask the countertransference of the analyst, that is, his preconceived idea about the patient. As a result, the Real with which the patient is dealing in analysis turns out to

[22] "It may be conceded that Sammy represents himself as a mouse, an animal cats play with. One can also suppose that the psychoanalyst is represented by a bottle . . . the child then introduces a bull which is evidently a symbolic representation of the father figure. The introduction of this symbol for the father is reassuring in view of the demands made by the little mouse on the mother (the bottle of milk), since the bull keeps separate the two figures of the subject and his psychoanalyst . . . this Oedipal situation, readily comprehensible to the observer, nevertheless has a very primitive character and employs very bizarre symbols, since the patient is represented by a mouse and the psychoanalyst appears as the object of the oral drives which are, as we shall see, highly important in Sammy. . . ." (Lebovici and McDougall, *Un Cas de psychose infantile.*)

be the analyst's fantasy world. This is a point that completely escapes the analyst; he has taken cover behind his cast-iron theory which can only remain infallible at the cost of condemning the patient to his status as patient. Two worlds are opposed: the world of the virtuous—the healthy—and the world of the guilty—the patient called upon to heal. The problem that lies at the heart of all analytic experience, namely, "Whom are we talking about? Who is talking to whom and on whose behalf?" is avoided altogether. The subject is never called upon to subjectively formulate in words the events of his past history. They are fixed once and for all in the analyst's mind as facts of development in which certain stages have been skipped. Preoccupied with the question of what course to take in regard to the subject, the analyst forgets to investigate his words.

In the analysis of Sammy's case,[23] the authors give us two separate texts—the child's words and the mother's during their separate treatments. The treatment was conducted as a dual relationship where the parents were merely listened to as purveyors of information. The authors do no more than mention the place occupied by the child in the mother's fantasy world although they note, very appropriately, that *the mother knew before the birth of her son* that she would get no pleasure out of him. Such a presentiment shows how important it is for the analyst to listen to the mother's word in the treatment of the child. Sammy was destined to be the mother's persecutory object even before his birth. From the outset, his mother situated him not in the place of the Other to whom one talks, but in the place of the Imaginary other, and in that dialogue there was clearly no room for Sammy; the mother—who included

---

[23] Sammy, a boy described as schizophrenic, was nine and a half years old when he entered psychotherapy in Paris with a new analyst—his third. He was an intelligent child, and we are told that he behaved aggressively towards a sister who was seven years younger. He was maladjusted in his behavior towards his classmates, children called him "crazy," and he was sent away from school after school for instability. Only a stay in a holiday camp did him good; here he made friends with a black child—a friendship categorized as "homosexual" by the adults. The child admired his father, who was a painter, but he obviously wanted to be punished.

Sammy, as her symptom—was self-sufficient. The adult left virtually no room in the child's life for desire which must always conform with that of the Other; thus we see the child struggling in a type of dual relationship where there is room only for one *or* the other of the partners. Yet, once again, it was on this ground plan that the analytic relationship was established.

The method of treatment paid no attention to a certain type of mother-child link; it was artificially focused on Sammy as the sole symptom, even though the mother was a partner in this symptom.[24]

The boy began the analysis with the "I" of a communication in which he asked a question relating to the desire of the Other;[25] failing to make himself heard on the themes that preoccupied him through this relationship with the Other (death; anxiety about being devoured),[26] he soon retreated to impersonal communication (the myth), or took refuge in clever, "grown-up" speech.[27]

The analyst's very conception of what was real and normal contained the clue which was to lead Sammy from the field of "reality" to that of a dual anxiety-laden relationship. Reality meant principally the analyst's fantasy world.[28] Sammy was inflexibly knocking himself against its walls, as he was doing at home against those of

[24] The difficulties started with birth—the baby refused the breast. A relationship of reciprocal rejection established itself between mother and child, which was subsequently expressed in the child in an insatiable and perpetually unsatisfied need to be loved. We are told that up to the age of nine he had been withdrawn into a dream world of his own, living with imaginary people, but one day the father forced him, "for his own good, to face up to reality," that is, give up fantasy stories (in effect, to change something at the level of words). The child loved to have his mother read him stories. One day it stopped; Sammy was too big for it.

[25] Sammy wondered what the analyst was going to do with his drawings. Did she want him to make her a present of them—or did analysis consist in integrating the drawings with what the child was saying?

[26] The child represented people by crosses in his drawings. Why were the living depicted by something that implied their extinction? (Sammy's father was Jewish but the child was never studied against the context of his background.)

[27] "There is a penis left behind in your vagina." "No," the analyst replied, "I haven't taken your penis."

[28] This brings us back to the problem of countertransference; the psychotic child arouses a form of primordial anxiety in the analyst, usually directed towards the mother.

his parents' intentions and expectations. Captive in the part he was playing, Sammy remained dramatically that even during analysis, sometimes attempting to reduce transference to the point where he was on his own, so as to have a protection against words he considered dangerous.[29]

Thus, at the beginning of treatment we witness the child's desperate attempts to remain sole lord of the fortress.

Next, we see Sam losing himself in a type of projected identification from which he could no longer escape.[30] The parents (it was mainly the mother's wish) decided, in agreement with the analyst, to put Sammy in a boarding school in America for psychotic children. The doctor at this establishment asked him to make three wishes. Sammy named "I want to be perfectly well when I grow up, I want to be the cleverest person in the world," and "I want to be famous."

The child wished to remain in his family; he tried to make his voice heard up to the end. "I wish my parents would ask me what I want to do, instead of going on with their own thoughts." No no-

---

[29] The analyst confused murderous (aggressive) *intent* with murder (aggression). But, Sammy lived in a fantastic-sadistic world where love was garbed in the same meaning as murder. This love (murder) was not directed towards the Other but towards the Imaginary other; it was thus suicide as much as it was murder.

[30] This process begins during the fourth session when the boy introduces the theme of the "magic face," which undergoes manifold changes until it disappears in death. (There is an *a-a'* relationship in this communication, which the analyst interprets as a relationship of the subject to the Other, thus making an erroneous intervention. See Jacques Lacan, "Du traitement possible de la psychose," *Ecrits,* p. 549.) "It went on bubbling away," said Sammy. "The sun got nearer and nearer, everything was dead, it was just the earth which went on turning around, all on its own. Everything was dead. Nothing but scorching earth and bubbling water. The earth got smaller and smaller and then, bang! bang! bang! the earth collided with the sun and there was a terrible explosion. Nothing remained alive. Then all that was left of the earth came out of the sun—it was just ashes. And that was the end of the earth. And there were only eight planets going around the sun instead of nine. It was very sad, what happened to the earth. There was only a tiny little bit of music left. Even the magic face was dead." The analyst adds: "In reply to my question, he said, 'You want to know too much. What would you do if the world really exploded?' He refused to say what he thought he or I would do in such a situation." (But, when Sammy said "you," he was not addressing the Other but merely an other.)

tice was taken of these words. It was a case of a misunderstanding, which prompts us to pursue our inquiries among the adults.

The symptom developed, of course, with and for an Other. The analyst thus became involved in the subject's speech. Sammy felt the need to put up the screen of his disorder between himself and the Other. He made his disorder the stake. Seductive and threatening by turns, he had his part—that of the mad boy. He had become the person who was spoken about, since he could not become the person who was spoken to. For whom should he speak when no one paid any heed to his desire? It was precisely as a boy alienated by the doctor's wish that he went to the institution in Chicago. Each protagonist in the drama situated himself in turn in the locus of the child (unhappy), in the place of the parents (who must be consoled) and of the adoptive mother (guilty of loving a child who had been cast out by his own mother). In the end, it was in fact Sammy's mother who conducted the game from the shadows. The father perceived this but, unconsciously, he did not want to know. It was probably for this reason that he needed an Other as prop for his belief—or his lie. "My son is psychotic, my daughter can't walk, and my wife is an alcoholic, yet everybody says that everything is fine. Perhaps it's just me who can't see straight. I intend to go and see Dr. B. *to find out* whether I'm nuts."

The father knew that the symptoms were alibis for a misfortune that had its seat elsewhere, but he could not discover the meaning because, each time, the symptom was objectified;[31] he left no room then for the word of the subject. The child became the anonymous pillar of a drama that was too big for him. In this world of deaf people, his words were destined to convey no message.

The interest of the book lies in its scientific objectivity. The authors display care, and courage, by providing a complete text rather than a method; the text invites a scrutiny of a technique. I became aware in reading it that it is a clinical approach which is the very

---

[31] The doctor satisfied himself with a relationship to the Real, which sometimes seems like self-justification.

reverse of ours. It is for that reason that I have stressed the methodological differences. For us,[32] analysis is not a dual relationship in which the analyst offers himself as the object of transference. The important factor is not the interpersonal relationship but what is going on in the process of communicating; that is, the locus *from which* the subject is speaking, *whom* he is addressing, and *for whom*. No interpretation can be made except by taking into account the register in which both analyst and analysand operate.[33] Without this, there is a risk of misinterpretation.

In 1907, Freud stressed that daydreaming is a form of play, and placed it in the transference relationship, remarking, "In some corner of the dream, just as the portrait of the donor is to be seen in many altar-pieces, there is a picture of the person to whom the dream is dedicated." It is in that "corner," in which transference has put us, that we receive the material the child brings.

Any interpretation in which the analyst is objectified destructures the subject; it does so to an even greater extent, if the analyst does not realize with which of the subject's promptings he is being identified at that juncture. Fantasy themes[34] are attempts at symbolization for the child; a myth often contains within itself the solution, the cure—as we saw in the case of Hans. Nevertheless, the themes, the signifiers, must still be brought out, not frozen by giving them the character of a literary production; otherwise, one will miss the chance of helping the subject to forge his truth[35] out of what is meaningless.

The approach in child psychoanalysis is by no means an easy matter; that is why we see so many differences of opinion on points

---

[32] I follow Lacan in this respect.

[33] Oral material must not be interpreted at a genital level, because if it is, it reinforces the subject's defenses—as happened in Sammy's case.

[34] Fantasy is a very precise story that can only emerge from anxiety, and it implies for the subject a threat from the Other, doubled by a danger of physical violence.

[35] By abandoning impersonal communication and becoming the subject in his words.

of technique. The range of techniques employed [36] (play therapy, relation therapy, release therapy, child guidance, etc.) is the measure of uncertainty among therapists. The child and his family pose a problem for the analyst. He feels himself exposed by the type of treatment he initiates.[37]

In 1927, Anna Freud restricted child psychoanalysis to those whose parents had been analyzed themselves, thereby revealing *her own need* to be understood by parents whose child she was unconsciously "stealing." Adherents to the Viennese school were the first to undertake analysis of children whose parents had not been analyzed, but they were careful to have frequent interviews with the parents. The introduction of the parents into the child's treatment became almost a rule for analysts in cases of children under five as well as in cases of psychosis. It is nevertheless striking to note to what extent they call upon the parents for assistance in *educational* matters as they intervene on the plane of *reality* in matters of family life.

This educational and social viewpoint has even led the British to establish a *child guidance* movement, which relies on a complete team centered around the child who is studied as a phenomenon. Different analysts look after the mother and the child; *the one looking after the child is thus cut off from the necessary contribution of the mother's words* and finds it difficult to take fantasy into sufficient account, since he is occupied with providing help in reality. Child psychoanalysis is regarded as corrective experience which the mother can subsequently continue on her own at home. The mother is coached by the analyst as to what she has to do—sometimes she has to apologize to the child for mistakes she has made. The analysts never stop delving into the place of the mother's words in the fantasy world of the child, as well as into the place of

[36] E. Buxbaum, "Technique of Child Therapy," in *The Psychoanalytic Study of the Child*, Vol. IX (1954).

[37] A.-A. Pichon-Rivière, "Quelques Considérations sur le transfert et contretransfert dans la psychanalyse d'enfants," *Revue française de psychanalyse*, Vol. XVI, Nos. 1–2 (January–June, 1952).

the father in the mother's words. And in prevailing on a mother to undergo analysis herself, instead of *hearing her while treating the child,* they do not reflect on the point that it is futile to analyze a mother on the basis of her own accounts, when her own accounts *are* the child to such an extent that her perpetual presence is expressed through the child's symptom. This reliance on reality is the hallmark of a school and a technique which fail with psychotic children. The only remedy considered for these is placement in an institution, in the hope that in the long run they will benefit from the influence of the environment. The Kleinian school, on the other hand, with its different theoretical conceptions, has been able to undertake the analysis of psychotics.

We shall see by examining certain works of English and American analysts that the problem of treatment, though correctly stated,[38] cannot be solved because of theoretical conceptions that produce misunderstandings and misinterpretations at the clinical level.

Dorothy Burlingham[39] relates the case of Bobby who was seen by different analysts at ages 2½, 3½, and 4½, for incontinence, anorexia, and speech retardation. Mother and child had instituted a *folie à deux* around the anal ritual by playing cat and mouse as the mother sang and caught her child's feces in a pot. Bobby entered into his mother's sadomasochistic setup, the parts being switched back and forth, we are told, as on the stage. The analysis of both ended in failure, which was attributed to the effect of the child's sex play with the mother. The father was never introduced into the treatment at all. What was singled out in the analyses was the overt attitude of the mother, but not her words. This theoretical position restricted the analyst in her listening and prevented the full use of the material she was given to interpet; also, the separate analyses of mother and child left unexplored the field where the words of

---

[38] The unconscious fantasy link between mother and child was obviously glimpsed at but not used in treatment. The mother's words, and what they implied in the various registers, were not taken into account sufficiently.

[39] Dorothy Burlingham, Alice Goldberger, Andre Lussier, "Simultaneous Analysis of Mother and Child," in *The Psychoanalytic Study of the Child*, Vol. X (1955).

mother and child were in fact constituted. We see the child in analysis hurling himself against the unconscious of the mother who, having already succeeded in outwitting the father, was now seeking to thwart the analysis of her child. It seems that the mother needed her son's analyst in order to introduce her word; not being listened to, she made her presence felt by the play of the symptom which she took pleasure in perpetuating. The failure of treatment is presented by the author as an inescapable fact; it never occurs to her to question the efficacy of the method.

Ilse Hellman[40] relates the analysis of a boy of eleven, conducted by two different analysts, one for the mother, the other for the child. The pathology common to both consisted in the mother's hypochondriac anxiety, expressed first in the somatic disorders of the child, then in his refusal to leave his mother to go to school. It was this symptom which led her to consult a psychoanalyst. The author shows us how the mother projected on her child her own relationship with her mother, a hypochondriac who had committed suicide. She could refuse her child nothing, for fear that he die. The link between the mother and her own mother, in all likelihood a homosexual one, created a situation from which men were excluded. The analysis is based on the *reality* of the mother's sexual assaults on her son, but her position in regard to *desire* goes unmentioned. We never get a hint at any stage of the part played by the father figure in her fantasy world. The analyst takes her at her word when she describes her husband as inferior to her and as having "a thumb missing," and never questions her about her own lack of being. In fact, the analyst echoes the woman's grievances; she also regards as "inadequate" the father who could not serve as a male identification for the boy. The analyst fails to distinguish between the person of the real father, and the place the mother assigned to him in her words. She listens to what is presented in the register of *demand* (lots of complaints), without realizing that what is being expressed thereby is connected to *de-*

40 Ilse Hellman *et al.,* "Simultaneous Analysis of a Mother and Child."

sire[41] (a wish to have an unfulfilled wish).[42] The mother's unconscious wish could not come to light in her own treatment, because the analyst had kept the interpretation at a level where the subject no longer had to orient herself in relation to the structure of her demand.

What goes unmentioned is the way in which the mother produced "revelations" about the "harm" she had been doing her son. She could not make these revelations to her son's analyst, because her words were not listened to there. Obviously, she uttered them elsewhere *so that they could get talked about,* and the analyst apparently failed to understand this verbal game. The fact that the two treatments were conducted separately made it impossible to understand the role assigned in the mother's fantasy to her son's analyst (as a third party); failing to be listened to in the quarter where her son took his symptom, she perpetuated her presence in his neurotic disorders. (In the mother's treatment, a certain method of analyzing resistances had made any unconscious "revelation" impossible, and lack of participation in her son's analysis barred the mother's access to a Symbolic dimension. In both cases, the mother remained under cover behind the organization of her defenses.) The harm admitted by the boy's mother was "real" and impressive —she had fed him "stale food," antidotes to poisons, even tablets for menstrual pains. The style in which the "poisoning" was carried out makes us see that it was in fact, *Imaginary injury,* with some support from reality, as the boy was hardly any the worse for it. Yet, each time, the meal was the starting point of a ceremony that was, above all, a *communication* in which the mother questioned the child about every conceivable illness that he might catch. It is obvious, although it escaped the analyst, that the mother was putting the questions to herself; in other words, the dialogue was not

41 J. Lacan, "Le désir et son interprétation," *Bulletin de psychologie,* Vol. XIII, Nos. 5–6 (January, 1960).

42 S. Freud, *The Interpretation of Dreams* (London, Allen & Unwin, 1954; New York, Basic Books, 1955).

in the least with a real Other—the boy—but with the mother's Imaginary other. Therefore, the "deadly" food has no meaning except *from its place* in the general context. This symptomatic communication (as it was subsequently reported) *also* occurred with the child's analyst, and it may be wondered how the authors could remain blind to it. The maternal communication could not but go on and on, because it achieved nothing. It was not regarded as the concern of the boy's analyst, although it reached him all the same through the boy's *words,* but we are left in the dark as to how the boy made use of his mother's words in the game that he himself was playing.

The boy's progress accompanied various illnesses and operations undergone by the mother, which resulted, I believe, from her failure to be heard by her son's analyst. Then an impasse was reached. The symptom persisted, as did a certain deceiving word of which the analyst had unwittingly made herself the accomplice.

In spite of the incontestable merits of these observations, it remains nevertheless true that a certain faith in positive explanations —in this case, an explanation based on "real" facts—brought about the obstruction of psychoanalytic insight, the result of which is felt in the conduct of treatment. This was carried on in a dual situation wherein the mother underwent treatment "for the good" of the child, without anyone ever stating to us what the child represented in her fantasy world. He was not only the object of her projections but also, and above all, served to mask her own lack of being. The mother could not accept her lack, and this was the source of the boy's inability to achieve structuralization outside her. The implications of this essential dimension were scarcely used in the treatment which kept strictly to the part played by the *real* penis of the child and the real food provided by the mother, and let slip away what the mother and child lacked at the *Symbolic* level. That route would lead us back to the castration problem in the mother and how it was presented at the level of desire, compelling the subject to take refuge in an endless search for demands.

When the subject's words are contrasted with "reality," the "true word" escapes to be replaced by deceiving words or a mask—the symptom that persists. The advent of the subject's word is thus jeopardized. As the result of their pursuit of *signification* (interpretation of symbols), the authors bypass the *meaning* in their treatment. The meaning can appear only by situating the subject's words more accurately in relation to his demand and his desire. Lacan[43] shows us what the subject who desires expects from the Other—he hopes to receive that which is lacking in his word. For the subject, the word constitutes a message. The hidden meaning is inscribed in the symptom. The subject is going to articulate a certain communication from the locus of the analyst. What he will *get back* will be his truth, which has been masked by illness or suffering. Viewed in this perspective, there is no *analytical dialogue,* there is only a vast utterance that begins in the locus of the Other and, moving forward, gains access to the Symbolic by releasing the subject from an Imaginary trap. Freud stressed the part overdetermination plays in the symptom. Lacan points out that overdetermination is conceivable only in the structure of language, and that all demands produce effects on the subject that vary according to the way he situates himself in a particular relationship to his fellowman. It is through language that he is going to break out of his Imaginary trap and articulate his demands, and do so with a mastery that he could not have attained under the influence of a purely Imaginary relationship. The subject's position in the symptom can be understood as the result of a failure of recognition in a certain

---

[43] J. Lacan, "La Direction de la cure et les principes de son pouvoir," in *Écrits* (Paris, Éditions du Seuil, 1966), p. 585. "Desire is what becomes manifest in the gap that demand hollows out beyond itself, to the extent that the subject, adding link by link to the chain of signifiers, reveals his lack of being and appeals to be complemented by the Other—if the Other, the locus of the word, is also the locus of this lack. Working through this again, the word is, first of all, a message for the subject, because it emanates from the locus of the Other. The fact that the subject's demand comes from the same source, and is labeled as such, does not mean only that is is dependent upon the code of the Other; it also means that it bears the dateline of the locus—and even of the time—of the Other."

type of relationship with the other. This shows how important it is that the analyst distinguish in his patient's words that which is addressed to the other (Imaginary) from what is said to the Other (the locus of the word); failure to do so lays him open to serious misunderstandings.[44] This is what happened in the cases of Sammy, Bobby, and Eric. Each remained fixed in the part of a "living puppet," and there remained fixed also the pathogenic parent to whom, through the symptom, each was attached.

As analysts, we find ourselves grappling with the history of a family. The direction treatment evolves in depends partly on our insight into a particular situation. The child who is brought to us does not come alone, for he occupies a definite place in the fantasy of both parents. As subject, he himself is often alienated in the desire of the Other. He cannot be isolated artificially from a certain familial context; from the outset, we must take into account the parents, their resistance, and our own. We too are implicated in the situation, with our own personal history; it is for that reason that we are able to find the meaning of the child's message, but also at the same time liable to resist it. A child's words (particularly those of a psychotic and mentally retarded child) always reveal a particular type of relationship with the mother. The child's "illness" constitutes the very locus of the mother's anxiety, a privileged anxiety that generally cuts across normal Oedipal development. The value placed by the mother on a particular type of illness transforms it into an object of exchange, creating a special situation in which the child attempts to escape from the father's domination. The "illness," which comes into being through the relationship of the child to the parents, imposes its component of anxiety in the first few months of the child's life. Also, it may not become a problem until after the

---

44 J. Lacan, "Direction de la cure." "This means that a subject's responses to a given demand are influenced by the effect of a particular position in relation to the other (here, 'the other' means another human being) which he maintains as subject. 'Which he maintains as subject' means that language enables him to see himself as the stage manager or even the producer of any Imaginary trap in which he would otherwise be only a living puppet."

acquisition of language or of motor autonomy. The mother's attitude induces a certain type of response in the child, owing to the fact that the child is physically and psychically deficient. A more thorough study might make it possible to explain the choice the child makes from among the various possible responses. When a physical factor is involved, the child is faced not only with an organic problem but also with the manner in which his mother takes advantage of this defect in a fantasy world that ends in being shared by both of them.

The reality of the "illness" is never underestimated in psychoanalysis, but an attempt is made to pinpoint just how the real situation is lived in by the child and his family. It is then that the symbolic value that the subject attaches to the situation, re-echoing a given family history, takes on a meaning. For the child it is the words spoken by those around him about his "illness" that assume importance. These words, or the absence of them, create the dimension of the lived experience in him. At the same time, it is the verbalization of a painful situation that makes it possible for him to bestow a meaning on what he is living through. Whatever the child's real state of deficiency or disturbance may be, the analyst endeavors to understand the words that remain petrified in an anxiety or encased in a physical disorder. In treatment, the subject's question will replace the demand or anxiety of parents and child, a question that is his deepest wish, concealed hitherto in a symptom or in a particular type of relationship with his surroundings. What will become clear is the manner in which the child bears the imprint not only of the way his birth was awaited but also of what he is going to represent for each parent as a function of their respective past histories. His real existence will thus come into conflict with the unconscious projections of his parents, and this is where the misunderstandings arise. If the child gets the impression that every access is barred to a true word, he can in some cases search for a possibility of expressing himself in illness. When parents and child are brought to face the problem of desire in the relationship of each of them with the

Other from the very outset of psychoanalytic treatment, the parents will be led to reappraise themselves in the context of their past history; and from the child, now addressed as the subject, the analyst will get words that are sometimes astonishingly articulate. This poses the question of language in a certain mode of relationship to the Other and to oneself. To abrogate words—which may be described as alienated in that they are the words of others and of general opinion—is a painful adventure for the subject. The analyst's job is to help him undertake it.

"The history of desire," Lacan tells us, "becomes organized in a style of communication which develops in the insane. This is the unconscious—in words wherein displacements and condensations doubtless correspond exactly to displacements and condensations in ordinary speech, that is, to metonyms and metaphors, but metaphors that—unlike ordinary metaphors—convey no meaning, and displacements that have no being, and in which the subject does not recognize something being displaced. It is around the exploration of this communication of the unconscious that our experience of analysis has grown." [45]

[45] J. Lacan, in seminar, May 13, 1959 (unpublished).

CHAPTER II

TRANSFERENCE IN CHILD PSYCHOANALYSIS: PRESENT-DAY PROBLEMS[1]

The discussion and controversy about whether or not transference occurs in child psychoanalysis is rendered difficult by the concept of transference adhered to by the analysts concerned. Their points of reference are affectivity, behavior, and adjustment, but these are inadequate to pin down what is really at issue.

I propose, first, to examine the manifestations of transference neurosis as they are described in two texts.[2] I shall deal with a particular juncture in the treatment. The common factor in the cases of Joy and Dottie is the manner in which analyst, parents, and child find themselves at a certain stage in the analysis drawn to the same field of play in an anxiety situation.

Joy, an eleven-year-old, suffered from pseudo-debility. The analyst demonstrates that it was the expression of an unconscious wish —the wish to have a penis, denial of differences between the sexes,

---

[1] Lecture to the *Schweizerische Gesellschaft für Kinder und Jugendliche,* Zurich, January 29, 1966. Published in *Revue de psychologie et des sciences de l'education,* preface by A. de Waelhens, Vol. I, No. 4 (1965–66). Also published in *Praxis der Kinderpsychologie und Kinderpsychiatrie* (May/June, 1967).

[2] Sara Kut, "Changing Pattern in the Analysis of an Eleven-Year-Old Girl," in *The Psychoanalytic Study of the Child,* Vol. VIII (1953). Selma H. Fraiberg, "Clinical Notes on the Nature of Transference in Child Analysis," *ibid.,* Vol. VI (1951).

and castration wishes, all associated with difficulties in arithmetic—which was to punctuate the various stages of transference and mark the child's early progress under treatment. Joy subsequently expressed oral demands in an increasingly regressive mode, although in real life she showed a thirst for knowledge alternating with a block against receiving it. The author describes a succession of forms of behavior which she calls *patterns*—in fact, role-playing. Joy *was* in turn her own father or mother, or husband or son of the analyst, even the analyst herself. This was reflected in her speech; she adopted her father's way of speaking or the slang of another child, a patient of whom she was jealous. She played the part of the analyst with younger children and even gave advice to mothers.

There occurred the *telephone episode,* which revealed the dynamics in play at a given moment in the transference situation. After Joy translated her jealousy and claims into transference, she expressed her wish to be "the only one." Since her parents were away—they had gone to the country because of a death in the family—the child was discontented. She made an admission to her analyst to the effect that she wished to fall ill so that her parents would be forced to cut their trip short. Soon thereafter Joy began to miss sessions and became more and more demanding. The analyst got the impression that she was seeking to revenge herself on the analyst for the abandonment into which she had been plunged by her parents' departure. When she came back after one of her absences, she let the analyst know about her bad state of health; she was on her own, and she was not feeling well. She contrived to alarm the analyst and extracted a promise to telephone her during the weekend to find out how she was. The analyst telephoned at the appointed time. She was told that Joy was out. That worried her and she called back a little later The child picked up the receiver but, seized by panic, she ran off. It took the analyst a while to realize that she was talking to thin air; there was no one at the other end of the line. Joy had disappeared. The next day, the girl notified her that she was going to miss a series of appointments.

Her return was accompanied by feelings of guilt. Joy felt herself to be one too many; she had the impression of interfering with an intimate meeting her analyst, who was unmarried, could be having with a man. Her schoolwork came to a halt. She was in a state of confusion. She could no longer do anything on her own. She *demanded* ideas from the analyst. She became more and more insistent, telephoning every day "to get an interpretation," until one day the analyst verbalized Joy's wish to have a baby. This was a turning point in the analysis. The girl turned out to be more intelligent than her mother, but her stealing, which was one of the symptoms, persisted.

The parents' *real* absence had given rise to an *Imaginary* injury, and the girl was endeavoring to compensate for it by making more and more insistent demands on the analyst. The interpretation bearing on Joy's wish to have a baby revealed the unconscious desire and, as such, was effective on the symptom level; she made no further demands. The analyst had nevertheless lent herself *in reality* to the telephone game, without trying to understand what factor was in play in Joy's demand for an interpretation. In questioning the analyst about desire for a man, the girl then introduced an element that both the analyst and she had lacked, in order to communicate completely outside the dual situation, that is, she was expecting the Other to redirect her complaints *elsewhere*. If the analyst's response was only partially effective, it was because what was in play in the anxiety of this appeal was something that was never tackled. The wish to have her father's baby merely paved the way to inquiries that should have been pursued but were cut short at this stage. Joy wanted to explore the workings of the Oedipus complex, but she lacked recognition points and so she turned her attention to what was involved in the analyst's desire. We see her becoming interested at a later stage in what the analyst was wearing, in her hobbies, her dates, her love affairs. She was clinging to *signs,* but that fact escaped the analyst who was maintaining her interpretation on the level of *behavior* (imitation of *patterns*), as if the child could be referred to satisfactions only on the level of Imaginary fascination. (It was on this level that the girl kept the interpretations she received; she did not take them up again in a second phase. The analyst's reply was *an* end, which was satisfactory in itself; it did not start new communication. And, in any case, the outcome of the analysis was conceived as identification with the superego of the analyst.) It was not at all surprising under the circumstances that the symptom of stealing persisted. The Oedipal problem remained unresolved.

In this fragment of the transference neurosis, the child's position in relation to her own desire and to that of the analyst was not explored at any time. Stress was laid on experiencing feelings and on imitating behavior patterns, but what was really in play in all this was left aside. If the Imaginary element of transference was glimpsed at, the Symbolic element went unmentioned, and it was on that level that Joy remained, as it were, stuck.

If Joy played a telephone game with her analyst, seven-year-old Dottie[3] fell prey to a dog phobia in the analyst's very house.

The day the child gave up the behavior disorder that had been the reason for her analysis, the mother had an attack of depression. Therefore, Dottie developed other symptoms, such as nervous tics, then fear of dogs. A phobic episode had kept the child from leaving the analyst's house for home on the very day when the mother telephoned the analyst, after the session, to tell her about the murder fantasies she entertained in relation to the child. "I'm afraid of what I might do to her," said the mother. The child had no knowledge of the 'phone call; she was in the waiting room where she had taken refuge after she had been seized by a fit of panic at the front door of the analyst's house. The mother's call made the analyst uneasy. She believed the child was in danger, and she thought that the mother ought to tell her own analyst about her fear. She did not realize that it was in the locus of the child's analysis that the mother needed to express her anxiety. Dottie herself was in tears;

---

[3] Fraiberg, "Clinical Notes on the Nature of Transference."

she did not even hear what the analyst said to her and merely answered, "I don't want to come back any more." The mother was depressed, the child was panic-stricken, and the analyst was worried because a third party, the mother, had invaded her relationship with Dottie.

Resistance is evident in *each* of the three participants. Each was afraid of the other. Each was under the Imaginary effect of a danger located in reality.

During a session in which Dottie expressed her desire to run out, the analyst, interpreting *this fear,* said, "Do you think I am a dog who will bite you?" and *barked.* The child, startled, began to laugh, and then we witness a real psychodrama wherein the parts are assigned and each in turn plays the dangerous dog for the other.

From the moment when Dottie identified with the aggressor, the phobic symptom vanished *on her trips to the analyst.* Within the transference, she was no longer afraid. Subsequently, the fear was localized elsewhere, and in due course it abated through the analysis of Oedipal material.[4]

One can see how the situation had come about. The progress of the analysis had led to a reactivation of the Oedipal situation in Dottie's family. She tried to defend herself against it, which translated itself in the transference as a resistance; the anxiety

---

[4] Dottie related a series of themes, including that of the *witch:* "A wicked queen got rid of her child, and the child ran off with her twin, who kept getting her into fixes. The children ran away, and the queen came after them. They finally took refuge with an old woman; lots and lots of children came to see her." *Sexual prohibition* appeared in the following form: "A boy and a girl were walking in the woods when they saw a sign saying 'Do not touch.' They touched it and were turned into statues. A prince rescued them, but the witch interfered again. On their way home, the children saw little statues of children turned into candy. So the children ate the candy, and the witch was going to eat them up. Only, she didn't eat them up, but they had to stay there for a year; then, when the year was up, they threw the witch in the oven." The analyst recognized the allusion to herself in this story. When the child started to get on to sexual problems she tried to escape analysis. She asked her father how much longer she had still to attend, and he replied, "For a year." The analyst noted that Dottie seemed afraid that something awful would happen to her if the therapeutic work drew closer to her sexual play.

thus induced was expressed in its turn by the sudden appearance of a dog phobia. It was at the father's request that the child had started analysis (the mother had been opposed to it), and Dottie's progress had a ravaging effect on the mother. Everyone in the family was in analysis with different analysts at that juncture. The day Dottie was taken in hand, a migraine symptom took over in the mother's case from the "child" symptom, which had been the persecutory object up to that point.

The analyst tried in vain to fend off the parents; in spite of herself, she found she was taking part in a collective utterance—child, analyst, and parents were all involved in one situation. It was in such a context that Dottie had to contrive to orient herself and throw off the Imaginary effects of anxiety and aggressiveness. But the analyst, although fearing that the mother might be dangerous, did her utmost to convince the child that reality was devoid of danger. There was no room in this analysis for the mother's fantasies; they were mentioned neither by analyst nor by child. Dottie, moreover, did not seem particularly worried about a real danger— she was occupied with an Imaginary fear in the shape of a dog. The stories she made up helped her find solutions to the fantasy effects caused by Imaginary aggression. Thus, the child's demands occupied the foreground and withstood all displacement (first, oral demands, then, seduction of father; she had offered to share his bed during the mother's absence).

It was a turning point in the analysis when she ran into the father's refusal (he declined the seduction offer in the name of the prohibition against incest). The child thereafter concentrated on orienting herself in relation to a triangular situation. She achieved it through myths, since they alone gave her that possibility of *symbolization* which was wanting in the analysis—as the analyst was unaware of the Symbolic element present in transference. What troubled the analyst in conducting treatment was the conviction that she was dealing with a mother who was harmful in *reality*.[5]

[5] "Upon closer examination, however, we find that this is not, properly speaking,

The admission of the mother's fantasies was always understood as a murderous intention and the mother's anxiety was discounted.

Now, it was really the Imaginary effects of her mother's panic to which Dottie was sensitive. The destruction fantasies of the adult endangered her, because in a primordial fashion they aroused her own fantasies about being devoured. Mother and daughter were thus involved in a transference situation. The mother, by her telephone call, was reminding her daughter's analyst of her presence, at the same time as Dottie, in her symptom, was giving evidence of her mother's unease. It was precisely in the locus of Dottie's analysis where each actor in the drama endeavored to make his words heard. The analyst, whether she liked it or not, was confronted with a collective communication. Mother and daughter were both wrestling with a form of anxiety associated with the fantasy nature of their projections. Each was a "dangerous dog" for the other; each brought her symptom to the analyst, as the third person, so that she could rid them of it (even if the mother appeared negative and the child pretended not to understand at all what was happening to her).

Lastly, the analyst herself was stamped by the anxiety or hostility of reciprocal transferences. She felt herself involved in the case— which, as far as misunderstandings went, assumed the proportions of a drama—to the extent of finding it necessary to defend herself by asserting that no transference had occurred. As we have seen, the analyst found herself confronted from the outset with the child's demands and the mother's complaints and claims. The risk did not lie wholly between mother and daughter, but also between child and analyst, because the latter feared that the child might prefer her to the mother.

---

a transference symptom. For the phobia originated in the child's relationship to her mother and maintained itself on this ground at the same time that it appeared in transference to the therapist. The transference of this symptom constituted a resistance against the therapeutic work. We could show Dottie that the therapist was not dangerous to her, but we could not yet deal successfully with the reality factors at home." (Fraiberg, "Clinical Notes on the Nature of Transference.")

In Dottie's analysis, transference was the expression of a defense position against anxiety at home, at school, or in analysis. The analyst failed to bring out the Symbolic element present in the transference situation, having reduced the idea of transference to a direct reference to her actual person. (Dottie found the solution to her phobia in myths.)

This case also shows that we have to deal with several transferences in child analysis (the analyst's, the parents', and the child's). The parents' reactions form an integral part of the child's symptom and therefore of the conduct of treatment. It is the analyst's own anxiety in face of the aggression or depression of the parents which usually leads him to deny the very possibility of a transference neurosis. The "sick" child forms part of a collective unease, his "illness" is the support of his parents' anxiety. In touching on the child's symptom, there is a danger of brutally laying bare the components that feed or, contrariwise, dam up the adult's anxiety. If the parent is given the idea that his relationship to the object of his care may be changed, defense and rejection reactions are aroused. Any suggestion that the child should be treated, even if there are realistically grounded reasons for it, challenges the parent, and child analysis can rarely be conducted without touching in some way on the fundamental problems of one parent or the other (their position with regard to sex, death, and the metaphor of the father). The analyst becomes sensitized to what is being expressed in these registers and takes part in the *situation* with his own transference. He has to define what the child represents in the fantasy world of the parents and at the same time understand as well the place the parents assign to him in the relationship he establishes with their child. If treatment is abruptly discontinued, it is usually because the analyst has failed to recognize the Imaginary effects on the parents of his own course with the child.

In the case of a *psychotic* child, parental anxiety is a continually recurring factor in analysis. It accompanies any step the child takes, forwards or backwards. Analysis of the child awakens the adult's own Oedipal problem in a brutal fashion. A mother who felt that she had no right to keep an Oedipal child sent her back to the destructive authority of her own mother, with the remark: "My father would be willing for me to get someone to look after Sophie, but my mother doesn't want it; she thinks that the child is all right only with her. She won't admit that she is ashamed of her. Sophie is abnormal, and my mother doesn't want the village to know about it, so she hides her." A father who was guilty of having an Oedipal child *sacrificed* him (and himself as well, in a need to make reparation): "I know that my son must die so that my daughter shan't be contaminated."

In a state of crisis, the parent is apt to blame the analyst—who gets downcast by it—and the child—whom he assaults in order to get at the analyst. "I've beaten him, I've scared him to death. But what do I count for you? I can burst, for all you care," one mother said to me, and the words—with slight variations—were subsequently re-echoed by the father of the same child! The words spoken to the analyst were death-wishes about the child. But the wishes were directed not so much against the parent's *real* child as against his Imaginary other.[6]

The Oedipal conflict that appears in this form—and is expressed in the transference situation in complaints, claims, or sacrificial offerings—conceals another, more complicated mechanism. The parent here puts himself in the *place* of the "sick" child, risking loss of his identity. "I'm as crazy as he is and in six months' time I'll kill myself," a father told me. At other times, a parent may compete with the analyst on the level of the Imaginary relationship which the latter is supposed to have established with the child. "That isn't what you should be saying to him!" a mother shouted at me, "After all, I'm in the best position to know what my child needs, I'm the only one who knows at that level. You can't take that away from me."

[6] The apparent danger of murder in fact conceals the danger of the parent's suicide.

What is in play in such dual mother-child situations is not confined to the child's relationship with the "pathogenic" parent, but also shows up in the transference situation. It arises as well in the special educational problem presented by the psychotic child, as the analyst discovers when he checks the work of the home teacher to whom he has entrusted the child. These are the various points that I shall now attempt to consider in greater depth.

The parents of six-year-old Emile were referred to me by the hospital, which had returned his medical file to them after having the boy for years of fruitless therapy. There was no doubt that the child had a condition of encephalopathy, but the sequelae were difficult to evaluate. The child did not talk and he became panic-stricken every time his mother left his sight. When he was four years old, Emile had let himself nearly die of hunger during a stay in the hospital; at five, he pined away in the same fashion when he was separated from his mother for ten months. "The case is one for the psychiatric ward," the parents were finally told, "but you can always try psychotherapy." I agreed to take the child for three months. A neuropsychiatrist encouraged me to do so; the medical diagnosis had, in fact, stressed the importance of the psychotic factor, but a psychoanalytic approach to the problem had been repeatedly ruled out because of the serious organic deficit. "Emile has been examined by so many specialists," his mother said, "but none of them even looked at him or spoke to him. A glance was enough. The one look crossed him off the list as a human being. They handed him back to us every time like a piece of scrap."

The mother was an intelligent young woman; Emile was her third child. It was because of him that she had given up work she enjoyed, to become a housewife by force of circumstances. The husband did not say much. He was marked by the burden of a seriously handicapped child. In his opinion the child was the victim of doctors and drugs. "Emile has been destined to be sacrificed. What can you do about it?" He saw no point in psychotherapy. Hadn't other doctors agreed that the child must be put away for the rest of his life? Why not get it over with? He was moved by his wife's distress, and she made a strong appeal to me for help. Putting the child away was postponed for three months. The father agreed not to make a possibly irreparable decision until a psychoanalytic approach had been tried. The mother had complete confidence in me at the first interview, but by the second she had changed her attitude and said, "And if nothing can be done, why not put him away at once? Then I shall stop thinking about it." Both parents were prepared to underwrite the hopeless diagnosis that had been pronounced. A reprieve was once more refused. I was astonished by this brusque change of mind. The child, whom I had not yet seen, was already in danger of being put away for good.

It was the parents' guilt that was expressing itself through the diagnosis they had seized upon. I said, "Anyone would think that you were convinced that Emile had no right to live, because the day you find people ready to help you, you give up. You even said you can't do that to Dr. X. But Dr. Y isn't trying to upstage Dr. X. He is simply asking to be given time before he states his opinion. It's you who are messing up the situation now by being in a hurry."

"First, they wanted to force us to try psychotherapy. Then, they said we could choose. It's not the same thing. We don't know about these things. Only the doctor *knows*," the mother insisted.

"The situation isn't clear," I said. "It was you who wanted your child treated 'like a human being'; those were your very words. The minute that becomes possible, you draw back, as if the psychoanalytic team, if it succeeds, were likely to do harm to the medical team which has withdrawn from the contest by its own admission. It is you, not the doctors, who are turning the thing into an alternative: either psychoanalysis—win or lose, you've turned your back on Dr. X—or putting Emile away at once—so as not to displease Dr. X who might turn nasty. You are ready to sacrifice Emile so as not to do him any harm."

"But what if his salvation lies in the Hereafter?" persisted the mother.

As she was leaving, she spoke to me in the same terms about her father. "He found his salvation in death"—in other words, by committing suicide. She was fourteen years old at the time. She tried in vain to resign herself to her loss by means of a condition of anorexia, which lasted several years. I pointed out the connection between the death of her father and that of Emile—not yet dead. The mother replied in tears, "They are like me; deep inside us we feel it an impossibility to live."

Here was a child who appeared to have no choice but to occupy as *subject* the place of a dead man. The seriousness of Emile's "illness" brought back for his mother both the anxiety aroused by her father's depression, and her own wishes to be done with life. For her, Emile was essentially a living being who was dead to other living beings, except to herself. "When he moves, I see my father in him." The fact that she had not resigned herself to her father's death had led the woman to resign herself to her child's death, though he was not yet dead—an act whereby she identified with her father. On the other hand, everything still prompted her to try to save him. "But have I the right to? What is going to happen to my other children?" What I was being asked to do was the equivalent of lifting an injunction. (An Oedipal guilt in connection with the child's "illness" had led the parents to state the chances of cure in terms of having a right to live.)

At the third session, I saw Emile with his mother. He was tiny, with huge, vacant, dark eyes; as soon as he was in his mother's lap, the eyes acquired an expression; at that instant he looked like a normal baby. He wandered round the room aimlessly, living everything inwardly. Emile not only did not play but was also unable to hold anything in his hands. If I went near him, he ran away. "You are scared I am going to take you away from Mummy. When you were separated from Mummy, you thought you were being punished for being naughty, and you were unhappy, but you couldn't find the words to speak your sadness."

The child climbed into his mother's lap and smothered her with kisses. "Poor little chap, he is getting on my nerves, I can't stand it any more," she whispered.

"Mummy is tired, but you haven't put anything bad in her. Sometimes it seems as if you were trying to be ill in Mummy's place."

The mother then recalled her anorexia, her fits of depression, and the fact that her husband's father had died when he was eight years old. "It was death that brought us together as husband and wife," she said.

In this fragment of the treatment, the following factors emerge:

1. The place I was to occupy in the transference situation from the outset; I was to be a miracle worker.

2. A series of dialectical *volte-faces: first,* the parents give up the idea of analysis and subscribe to the original diagnosis "in the child's interest"; *second,* the place reserved for the child (that of being dead), is brought into play re-echoing the Oedipal problem of the parents; *third,* the mother "feels" the child—she could play a beneficial role in the psychotherapy. "But have I the right to?" she then asks herself, as if the child's getting better ran counter to some sort of taboo.

3. The start of psychoanalytic treatment with mother and child. The child responds by the language of his body, by moving away from or closer to his mother. The mother then finds words to recall memories centered entirely around her uncompleted mourning for her own father.

The parents embarked on the course of treatment with a demand which they subsequently tried to cancel. The desire they imputed to me—to cure their child—aroused their problems about prohibitions. The question being asked in transference was fundamentally this: Oughtn't we allow Emile to die (thus fulfilling what we consider to be his destiny) rather than force him to live? The parents hoped that I would be the one to pontificate on the choice.

In her communication the mother occasionally put herself in the place of death (out of identification with the lost object?); when she made an appeal to me, she had to unmake it later, as if a sort of panic had been driving her so that she could never stay on the level of what she desired. When she desired herself to desire her son to get well, the problem of death arose (her father's, her son's, and her own), as if she had been nostalgic for an impossible past that Emile had the task of keeping alive.

All serious organic illnesses in children leave their imprint on the parents in ways that depend on their own past history. This became apparent in the transference situation in this case.

Let us re-examine the situation. In the transference of Emile's mother towards me there was a Symbolic element and an Imaginary element. She knew even before her son started treatment that she could expect any outcome from analysis, including the most bitter disappointment. Thus the reasons for breaking off treatment had been collected before I arrived on the scene. It was to the extent that I was the embodiment of a certain knowledge and the representation of a magic omnipotence on the fantasy plane of the parents, particularly, of the mother, that our encounter in reality precipitated a sort of *acting-out* (decisions to break off treatment) in accordance with a pre-established unconscious process. The transference thus existed *before* the appearance of the analyst. The countless medical consultations, the husband's interventions, the suggestion of putting the child away—first entertained, then rejected—all these were effects of the mother's anxiety. It was the mother who pulled the strings in a game where everyone else soon found himself outclassed. She induced the contradictory medical opinions and threw those who were looking after the child into a panic. She thus found in reality confirmation of her belief that she could not expect anything from anyone; as soon as she had found a chance of not being let down, she began to manipulate things so that nothing should be achieved.

Treatment was not broken off only because of the presence of an *Imaginary* element in the transference. I was seeing the mother and child together in sessions, and the feeling she derived from being regarded by me jointly with the child (whom others regarded as scrap) enabled her to find it possible to reinvest in herself as subject on a narcissistic level. She formed a single whole with that lost being, and I spoke to that single whole. The child responded to my interpretations with body movements, the mother recalled the past in words and wept. She found in me an ideal support for making it possible for her to accept herself, even to esteem herself, as a "good mother." Also, in the relationship there was something present as a ternary point of reference, therefore something Symbolic, since our relationship was governed by rules that served to help in curing her son.

In all this, transference was not merely the outcome of interpersonal relationship. As we have seen, a scenario had been worked out beforehand, one in which the reasons for breaking off treatment were laid out. I could not unmask the deceptive nature of this scenario, except by understanding that the mother had situated her truth within it. We could not be helped by analyzing her resistances, but only by bringing to light what was in play in her relationships to sex, death, the metaphor of the father—in other words, to that which had mattered for her on the level of desire in various forms of identification. (We have seen the part played by the unconscious correlation of her father's death, her own suicidal ideas, and the acceptance of the death of a child who is still alive.)

There is some connection between the questions regarding transference raised by this case, and the difficulties experienced by Freud in the analysis of Dora. Even before Dora entered analysis, she had sketched out in a dream the place to be reserved for Freud in transference. But Freud was looking for pointers to his place in Dora's associations of ideas, hoping to find there signs of resistance or to recognize forms of displacement, and transference never appeared where he thought he was going to find it.[7] In that period of his

[7] Dora's analysis can be partially described as the unfolding of her dream fantasy, transference being expressed on two levels. First, the girl placed herself in an Imaginary relationship with her father and polarized her interests on all the women who caught his attention. That was the context of her question about what she was.

career, Freud could not know that he was to run into a scenario where everything had been worked out beforehand, including the failure of his intervention.

Emile was three years old when certain doctors stressed that the psychotic factor was aggravating his organic deficiencies, but the mother's attitude had discouraged any psychoanalytic approach to the problem. Her claims about the medical profession had no other purpose than to announce from the rooftops the powerlessness of all doctors. Yet, that was the very element that was subsequently to nourish the transference which existed even before the mother met me.

It is essential to understand this situation, because it is the model of a type of *mother-doctor* relationship in which the child is used to underline the inadequacy of the doctor. But, the game of analysis is played on another level as well. The work of analysis must start in the pathogenic *mother-child* relationship, and not just in exposing the dual relationship but in introducing it, for what it is, into transference. It is through doing this that we help the mother first, redirecting her to narcissistic investment; then, in a relationship with the other the third element (signifier)[8] arises, enabling the mother

---

Second, through the list of demands presented by Dora, it was clear that she was seeking to receive her truth from the locus of an Other, but it was ordained that men were bound to fail with her. Freud discerned that element only after the decision to break off treatment. (One finds that decision running like a fine thread through the whole performance put on by Dora. But Freud had not yet grasped the part played by the Symbolic element in transference in that period.) Cf. J. Lacan's seminars on January 9, 16, 23, 1957. Report by J.-B. Pontalis in the *Bulletin de psychologie,* Vol. X, No. 10 (April, 1957): "La Relation d'objet et les structures freudiennes."

[8] *Signifier* (unit of the code): The term is borrowed from de Saussure, employed in a concept where the unconscious is regarded as being structured like a language (Lacan). One aspect of the speech of the unconscious, as Freud stressed, is that it is in obedience to strict laws that the effects of the displacement (*Verschiebung*) and condensation (*Verdichtung*) mechanisms appear in the speech of the subject. Interplay between meaning and literal meaning takes place on the level of unconscious speech. Association of ideas occurs on two tracks, the literal track being termed "signifier" and the meaning track "significant" (cf. J. Laplanche and S. Leclaire, "L'Inconscient," *Les Temps modernes,* July, 1961). The condensation mechanism results from substituting one signifier for another, producing a metaphorical

to orient herself—that is, to situate herself by relating to her own fundamental problems without including the child in them any longer.

Dora's treatment was compromised from the outset because, for one, she entered into it at her father's request. The father expected that Freud would become the accomplice of his deception, and Dora, sensing this, repeatedly stressed her father's "insincerity and deviousness." It was not irrelevant to Dora's subsequent simultaneous desertion of the K's, Freud, and her father, but not before she had regained the "right" of knowing that she was being lied to, as well as the pleasure of loudly proclaiming the fact to everyone's embarrassment.

Parental demands that a "sick" child be cured must be situated first in their fantasy level (particularly the mother's),[9] and then understood on the child's level (Does he feel affected by the demand for his cure? How is he using his "illness" in his relations with the Other?). The child cannot co-operate willingly in analysis unless he is assured that it is serving his own interests and not those of the adults.

The same problem arises, though in a different fashion, in cases of psychosis and retardation. When mother and child are in a dual relationship, it is in the transference that we can study the play of this relationship and construct interpretations of the manner, for example, in which the child's needs are perceived by the mother. It is here that certain fundamental positions of the mother are touched on, which often can be analyzed only through anxiety and in a persecutory situation.

The treatment of Christiane (a six-year-old psychotic girl)[10] was nearly brought to an end by the mother when I encouraged her

---

effect. Displacement, on the other hand, is the linking of one signifier with another, and has a metonymic effect. As any analysis proceeds, the "key signifiers" (death, phallus, Name of the Father, etc.) appear.

[9] What the signifiers "child" and "sick child" mean for her.

[10] When I refer to treatments for which I have been personally responsible, the *diagnosis* has always been made by one, or even two or three neuropsychiatrists. The children have been referred to me in the light of the diagnosis.

educator's[11] desire to take the child home with her during the holidays. The mother, whose attitude towards me had been positive, suddenly felt herself in danger of being rejected, or rather supplanted. In a real frenzy of anxiety, she asked her husband to stop the abduction of her daughter which was, in her view, being plotted. This *acting-out* was associated with my words, quoted by the educator to the mother ("Mme. M. agrees with my suggestion, what do you think?"). I had been rash enough to approve a suggestion before I had made its meaning clear to the mother. What was unacceptable on a Symbolic level was lived on the level of an Imaginary injury. Thus arose the fantasy in which daughter was torn from mother who could not live without her; and so, suffering intense emotional upset, she called on her husband for help. He must intervene *so that her child be left with her.*

The meaning of this demand was made plain in the reproaches she addressed to me: "Do you want my daughter to stop going to the bathroom, stop eating, and risk drowning?" These words were said in the presence of the child who witnessed her mother's confusion in panic, and responded to what was a situation of anxiety by becoming constipated. The mother countered this refusal on the child's part by begging her in tears, on her knees, "Will you give me *my* doodoo?" She became more and more insistent and finally, beside herself, she screamed the ultimate threat at her: "If you don't give it to me, I shall come and take it out of you."

During a session Christiane mimed a devouring mother who forces the baby to hand over her eyes, her mouth, the hole in her behind, the hole in her front, the holes in her ears, the holes in her nose. The baby in the game of mime ended up by losing itself in a *symbol*[12] offered to the mother.

The danger of the transference situation became evident to

[11] The term "educator" has a special meaning in the French educational system. See footnote 7 in Appendix I.

[12] What was extracted from the various parts (nose, ears, intestines) was the orifice, and as such it was taken as representing the maternal function; it is in this sense that I call it a "symbol."

Christiane when her mother lost the recognition points of her own identity in her panic. To avoid the risk of being abandoned, Christiane, in response to her mother's confusion, made herself into a mouth to be fed and an anus from which stools were removed—and in her play she demonstrated that she had lost herself as subject.

At the following session, Christiane was total refusal. The analyst, by having put the mother in danger, destroyed the relation to the third party that had existed in the mother's Imaginary transference.

It was possible for the mother to be a therapeutic agent so long as I maintained Christiane's presence in reality. She was seeking to gain value in my eyes as a good mother in her relationship with the child, by restraining her demands so that Christiane would succeed in being born to desire. She situated herself in relation to my desire, in order to be able to accept a situation where Christiane no longer filled her lack. But she could do it only if she felt herself narcissistically invested by me as mother. Transference opened up for her the possibility of desexualizing her links with her daughter, and it helped her discover tenderness: "Seeing you with Christiane has changed my attitude towards her." The mother had found a prop in her relationship with her child through the intermediary of the image of the other's body. It was because I had minimized (or refused) the overwhelming extent of her transference that I made the mistake of approving a separation just at the time when the child was beginning to come out of her psychosis. The upset that followed made itself felt beyond the mother, at the child's level, as she was assailed by a mother who had suddenly lost all identification. The repetitive factor in the transference situation was the pattern according to which the child regressed in the forms demanded of her, until she confined herself to being merely a mouth or an anus. The mother's panic was brought about by words heard and repeated by the educator, although at the level of what was signified, my remark was not in the least alarming. Why shouldn't the child go off with her educator? I had issued no orders about it. The mother reacted to a feeling of danger that already existed at the unconscious level, and the educator's words had merely given substance to a pre-existing fantasy. In this fantasy, the mother, as subject, held on to the child whom people wanted to tear away from her (as in a sort of Imaginary fascination). In reality, the young woman changed into a screaming mother who wreaked terror. A very precocious anxiety situation was being relived in the transference. The mother felt herself persecuted in imagination, pursued by the fantasy figures of her parents who desired her destruction. All of a sudden, she had no one to whom she could refer herself. The incident provoked a depersonalization crisis, and it was only afterwards that I learned from the mother what she had wished to keep from me: "I had an insane father who was confined for paranoia, and later sent back to his family. My mother was a screamer. Between the two of them, I was completely dazed. When I was fifteen, I had a nervous depression. Then I got TB. I was ill every time when my older children were born, but I got my health back with Christiane's illness. I spent my time on her and not on myself." [13]

Transference in this case was not established, however, by the sole direct relation to my person. Unconscious elements were in play, arousing an anxiety situation concerned with an Imaginary danger in which I had been cast from the outset as an agent of castration. The conflict was lived as a sort of transfer of title, with the husband now invested with the emotions formerly expended on the analyst. The role of healer now passed to him, and because he had not been involved in a persecutory situation, the analysis of the mother-child pair could continue. Later analysis of this incident in the treatment showed that the mother had appealed to her husband to insure that nothing change, in other words, that she remain in charge of the game. (The analysis of the child brought to light the mother's difficulties in her relationship to the law; to be marked by the law

[13] These words illuminate the way in which Christiane's body could become her mother's second body: "Will you give me *my* doodoo?"

referred her to the insanity of her own father, and she refused to be a toy in the hands of a capricious law. She fastened on the signs of this caprice in the attack of panic that seized her in transference. But, one might say that she had been expecting these signs from the time the child started treatment; that is the important element.)

Christiane responded to the dangerous situation of transference by effacing herself as subject of desire and becoming a pure symbol —an offering to be made beyond the mother, to the dead. She reproduced the response that she had always made to her mother; although analysis had jolted it into another register, the mother's reactions induced the child to efface what had been acquired. Her mother's desire was precisely that Christiane should not be born to desire. (The Wolf Man was also blocked at an early age by death in the desire of the Other; Freud throws light in this case on the unconscious wish of the patient to know nothing, not only about the castration problem but also about all forms of desire. The denial went so far that we see the subject disappear into his fantasy constructions.) After making spectacular progress, Christiane went through a regressive episode in transference; she rejected me and expressed her wish to remain in a state of non-desire, in response to her mother's persecutory position. She reproduced the obsessional ceremony that had marked the beginning of her treatment: she removed all traces of dirt, footprints, and smudges, and only after she had completely cleaned a particular circular space did she take up her position in it. The child obviously felt herself in danger of being attacked by me, as her mother had; to avoid any trouble, including being caught in a sandwich between her mother and myself, she was prepared to remain permanently petrified in her psychosis. Her games became increasingly stereotyped; she whispered with a faraway look in her eyes, repeating over and over again, "All gone, hole." It was her corpse that she was giving over to me. The day her mother "recovered," the child buried herself in my lap in the mother's presence. In a game, I gave her a feeding-cup, referring thereby to what she had once received from her mother. It was also by my referring, in words, to her having once lived in sharing her mother's body that the child could trust herself further in the adventure of analysis, in agreement with the mother who no longer feared that I was going to kidnap her child. Analysis of the negative transference in patients of this type, and of their mothers, brings to light the fantasy side of their emotions. Christiane refused to get well if her mother was to die as a result of it. It was only a long time afterwards that the mother was able to explain exactly the factors that were in play during her panic: "The revelation of my jealousy and hatred hit me full in the face, and in the same flash I had to come to terms with her being taken away. I can't explain any more. All I do know is that you had the power to drive me mad."

The mother could establish a relationship of trust only by way of a breaking point; therein the narcissistic component she had been able to invest in me simultaneously disappeared and was retained. I could have avoided the break. It occurred only because beneath the surface of her love towards me there lay hidden "a hatred" and unconscious death-wishes. The educator's words served merely to connect what was already inscribed in her unconscious; the fusion produced the intense emotional effect. A remark she made at the start of treatment, "Professor X trusts no one but you, and as for me, I know you'll make Christiane well," had a corollary in another phrase—the full significance of which became apparent only later on—"You'll fail, too, like the others [meaning, those men]. Christiane has only me to count on." Her resistance, when it took the form of hostility towards me, was in effect but the obstacle in her own language against recognizing an unconscious desire. The fantasy of the child's kidnapping had no purpose but to veil what she wished to keep hidden from herself. Her words (exactly as in the case of the Wolf Man[14]) were disturbing to the child, be-

14 For Freud, the revealing factors were the mother's words, the effects of the unsaid on a human destiny, and the fashion in which all sexual curiosity was prematurely foreclosed in the Wolf Man (i.e., any position of the subject towards

cause they played a decisive role through the chances of identification[15] they offered or refused her.

I have described[16] how Leon, a psychotic four-year-old, was affected by the words and silences of his mother. The effects did not go so far as to cause *trauma* in the limited sense that the term is generally applied.[17] (The panic effects of trauma bring about regression, even fixation. From this base, the subject, in a desperate search for the Symbolic dimension missing from the real event, attempts to implant substitute signifiers in himself.) Generally speaking, what occurs more frequently is *a block in the access to desire* for the child, with a quasi-injunction against revealing himself as other than alienated in his mother's wishes. Thus a situation arises in which the child feels himself to be on his own (through the effect of non-meaning created by the mother's words), without any possibility of introducing an Imaginary dimension,[18] lacking as he

---

desire). The Wolf Man was to his old Nanny the substitute for a son who had died very young. It was in the likeness of that dead child that he maintained himself in his desire. He was blocked in by a depressive father and a mother preoccupied with abdominal pains ("I cannot go on living like this"). He did not detect any desire to live in the adults. He was desired by the Other to be without desire, and he became petrified in non-desire between the ages of four and five.

15 *Identification:* In *psychoses,* the mother's words (which subtend the mother's fantasy) make it impossible for the child to maintain himself, except on the level of demand, never attaining the possibility of object identification. In *neuroses,* on the other hand, the mother's words refer the child to possibilities of identification, but conflicting ones.

16 See Appendix I. Leon was isolated in a pure state of non-meaning and could materialize his emotion only in a corresponding attack of epilepsy. Stamped by his mother's drama, he remained alone with his image, a prey to total panic, for want of an Other to whom he might refer.

17 *Trauma:* The intervention of a painful event in reality, the arbitrary occurrence of which leaves the subject unable to extract meaning on the symbolic (metaphorical) plane because it was not transmitted along the signifier track (cf. S. Ferenczi, "The Psychic Consequences of a Castration" in *Further Contributions to the Theory and Technique of Psychoanalysis* [London, Hogarth Press, 1951; New York, Basic Books, 1952]).

18 *Imaginary dimension:* Since the identification procedure is unconscious, the subject cannot know with whom he is identifying. His question about what he is, is asked from the locus of the Other. It is the *look of the Other* which reflects back to him the image of what he is. Recognition points of identity become lost

does the mother's mediation in the form of a meaningful word. This mediation is necessary if the child is to accept his own image. I attempted to introduce this Imaginary dimension into the treatment by the subterfuge of language.

Transference was established with the child when a correct interpretation cut short a fit of anger and stopped an "epileptic absence." Leon's previously suicidal behavior during sessions was foreclosed by the transference. Even if he could not establish an Imaginary relationship with me, I existed and spoke from a locus where truth compelled recognition. I broke a narcissistic relationship whose outlet was self-destruction or the destruction of the Other, by introducing from the very first session the conceptions of Leon's body and the Other's body, Leon's existence and his father's existence, Leon's existence and his mother's existence. The immediate effect was to cut short a fit of anger in which the child was trying to injure himself. The mere fact of saying "This is Leon's body, that is the Gentleman, Leon and the Gentleman aren't the same" made it possible for the child, and for his mother, to begin analysis. The mother established an Imaginary relationship with my person which enabled her, first, to be a "good mother" to the child under my supervision (at such times, what she said had meaning); and second, to shift to the locus of the Other as the source of truth (on a Symbolic level). She provided a commentary on the interpretations which I gave the child.

"It's the first time a tantrum has stopped short like that. I noticed you told him that the Gentleman isn't him. That must be an important point. As far as I'm concerned, I see and hear nothing but him, and I scream at him till he just gets me to the end of my rope."

In working with the child I introduced, in the mother's presence,

---

when the child cannot take hold of himself in the look of the Other, because the unconscious desire of the Other which subtends this look is felt to be a desire for death. The subject finds it difficult thereafter to establish an Imaginary relationship. We also find the absence of an Imaginary dimension in some forms of psychosis.

what was lacking in his relationship with his mother, situating him systematically in relation to his parents. My place was *elsewhere,* beyond human beings; it was actually the "magic" of the word that acted (like an oracle) on the child and his parents. It did so by introducing an axis (the phallus) around which the parents could question themselves about their relation to death, to the metaphor of the father, etc. The child's spectacular improvement (he recovered the ability to sleep, regained motility, the epileptic attacks ceased, and he began to use words) did not take place on a relational plane. What I changed were the structures[19]—it was with his educator and his mother that the change on the relational plane was to be accomplished, but only after a complete shake-up in both parents whose own recognition points had been challenged. The outward signs of transference were of two types:

1. The parents sought to understand their own anxieties and depressions, with reference to their own history. They had a positive attitude towards me and each related what had gone wrong in them on the Symbolic level.

2. Or, in an Imaginary relationship with me, they felt I was persecuting and bullying them, and struck at the child in an almost murderous manner. Leon, regarded as a bad object, was rejected; he was a piece of junk offered for my inspection in such a way as to make me unhappy, because the parents were touching on something that was at the level of the good interiorized object in my transference on Leon. It was important not to give in to a persecutory reaction, attacking the parents in my turn, because it was but a child-parent rivalry on the Imaginary plane in which I was the stake. The rivalry was expressed in the form of a choice: life or death for Leon, or for his parents. That was the alternative constantly put before me. It was essential never to take these reactions on the level of reality by yielding to the temptation of investment, but on the only level where it was possible to do something con-

---

[19] My aim was not to normalize the relationship of the child to myself but, as it were, to language.

structive, i.e., the analytic dimension. In this dimension, I was dealing with the Oedipal drama of both parents. The communication was a collective utterance, and the child appeared in it at an early stage, as the parents' Imaginary other. It was not surprising therefore that the parents experienced persecutory and depressive reactions on the transference level to the extent that the child began to exist otherwise than alienated in them. It was by keeping myself on a Symbolic level [20] that I was present for Leon. "The name of Madame Mannoni has a magic power," the mother said. "Just by saying it at home, we get the child to obey."

One day, in the mother's presence, I introduced the following notions in regard to a food phobia—the child refused to sit through the meal of an Other; seeing someone eat sent him into convulsions.

1. Leon has the sexual parts of a boy. He cannot desire to be Daddy's or Mummy's sexual parts.

2. You must not be afraid when you eat, because you are not the meat that is being eaten. Human beings are forbidden to eat each other. You have the sexual parts of a boy. You are not a tasty little morsel to eat.

These remarks introduced the idea of the anthropophagic taboo,[21] and cured the phobic attack. However, I provoked prostration in the parents; the fact that I had brought the signifier "phallus" into play with the child referred both parents back to their respective relations to their Oedipal problem, and produced aggressiveness

[20] It was by making apparent in words what remained unrecognized in the mother's desire (namely, to know the desire of the Other) that the dimension of a subject who speaks in the collective adventure was introduced in the child; i.e., of someone governed by the law of language where the word breaks an effect of non-meaning. The subject, through the mediation of the word of the Other, may succeed in introducing the Imaginary dimension, of which he has been deprived.

[21] *Anthropophagic taboo:* If, at the Oedipal stage, there is a *taboo against incest* that plays a structuring part in the development of the subject, then, before Oedipus the *anthropophagic taboo* (prohibition of parasitic action) plays the same structuring part. This also implies a reference to a third element, i.e., to the Law of the Father. It is of fundamental importance to highlight this idea in the treatment of psychotics.

towards me at the child's expense. Each time, there was a surge of emotion (one parent or the other was suddenly alienated in fantasy), but after a single interview they could speak to the child again, for the parents' depression was played out on the plane of the word which could only be deadly.

In effect, what we were witnessing was this: The child (feeling in danger of being eaten) fell prey to a persecutory anxiety which he sought to fend off by attacking the father, who compensated for it by turning on the mother. A serious quarrel ensued between father and mother which the child perceived as the re-enactment of the primal scene and lived through as a murder; it provoked suicidal reactions in the child who "mutilated" himself, and it ended with the parents' bringing a blood-stained, screaming child to the analyst, as demented as he had been on the first day.

On the technical level, interpretations were made in two contexts:

1. *The child in his parents' presence.* The confusion was cleared up by insisting on the fact that Leon's body and the Other's body were not the same—by giving a name to a danger localized outside the child.

2. *In separate interviews with the parents.* I listened to their own depression or more precisely, to what was functioning in them as a bad internal object (in their case, a real labor of mourning—mourning for their relationship with a dead parent). Leon, in his relationship with each parent, was put in the place of one dead, making it impossible for him to be the subject of any desire.

Treatment was conducted by the interplay of reciprocal transferences. What was emphasized was not so much the object relationship as the place of desire in the subject's internal economy, and this was highlighted by transference. (In Leon's case, one had to consider the position of each participant in the face of incestuous desire, anthropophagic desire, and so on.)

Work on the structural plane in analysis with a psychotic child brings about an improvement on his relational level with parents and educator, but the adult always has to pay some sort of price when a seriously disturbed child gets better. I think that the reactions of three educators to the progress made by a demented child are very instructive on this subject.

Sophie was five years old and had been diagnosed as "insane." Confinement in an asylum was deemed advisable. Subject to encopresis, enuresis, and epileptic fits, the child was in the grip of a total panic that revealed itself in destructive gestures. No human identification was possible; Sophie appeared to be concealed by a mask,[22] but behind the mask was yet another mask. She situated herself between the two. To the extent that she counted to herself at all, she was neither one nor the other. Every time the problem arose for Sophie to appear as a girl without a mask, that is, to be born as an object of desire, she was seized by panic because she might then count to herself, which meant that she would perceive her own lack. To perceive one's own lack is a problem of living as an echo of the problem of one's mother or her substitute.

When an educator was engaged for Sophie, the mother had a fit of depression: "I don't know what to do with my spare time. I keep thinking about Sophie, about what may happen. I was so used to Sophie's taking up all my time during the day that I didn't even have to think. In the evening with my husband I am a different woman, but I am not really there. Now she has an educator, I am lost, and I don't know what to do. I can't keep up a conversation any more. I miss Sophie."

The educator, Bernadette, was formerly schizophrenic. She had not finished her analysis but had substituted courses of study instead, and become an educator of retarded children. She was taken on by the family because at that time no one else would agree to

[22] The child disguised herself in a variety of penile substitutes, and finally became the emblem of the father as excrement, which incarnated the unthinkable side of birth. Sophie either felt herself to be loved as something-lacking-to-her-mother (and it was impossible for her to be), or else she did exist but ran the danger of being shut out (and could only maintain herself on the level of flight, epileptic fits, or total destruction of everything surrounding her).

look after such a fiendish child. At the outset, her presence was beneficial; she masked her fear by presenting herself to Sophie as an object of persecution. Bernadette became Sophie's thing. Sophie could choke her or defecate on her, and Bernadette would remark, "You see, we are fond of each other." I realized that the situation might prove to be upsetting to Bernadette, but she was "coping," as they say, and I could not but continue with a hazardous experiment. Bernadette wanted to keep her job. Sophie's mother had got used to her, and her father did not want to know anything about Bernadette's difficulties. ("We would never find anyone else to put up with what she does.") Bernadette told me about herself in talking about Sophie: "It is as if I were continuing my analysis with you," she said; "while I am with Sophie, you don't leave me, and that's what makes me feel safe." On another occasion, she said, "Sophie's mother has everything, really—a husband, money, and a daughter. I have nothing. I am having the most bizarre dreams which keep coming back. I am on a sandwich. The mother is outside and Sophie is a flower. The mother shuts us in. I feel I am in danger. It isn't easy to look after children like that. You get caught up in their own game without realizing it. There are times when I am scared I'll behave like Sophie. I get a grip on myself because I am an educator."

Bernadette managed to keep going for three months by means of an Imaginary reference to myself; then she complained that I was letting her down. From that time on, Sophie's mother seemed to be dangerous to her and in terms of their relationship on the fantasy plane it would have been difficult to say which one ran the greater risk of being devoured by the other. Sophie's "illness" became the stake in the relationship of educator to mother, and of educator to myself. "If Sophie didn't exist, you would have no further interest in me." One day, drama intervened. Sophie had an epileptic fit in the street. Bernadette ran off, found Sophie's mother at home, and said to her, "I am ill, I want to go to bed."

"But where is Sophie?" asked the mother.

"I have no idea where I left her—I have had enough of it. It doesn't matter what happens to me, only Sophie matters to you."

During the morning of the same day, Sophie stood in front of a mirror. "That's not Sophie," the child said to Bernadette. "You understand, don't you, that there isn't any Sophie any more."

"Why not?"

"Don't you understand that there mustn't ever be any more Sophie, ever! There isn't any more Sophie. It's Bernadette now. You see," the child stamped her feet, "Sophie flew away into Bernadette."

"My problem," Bernadette had been saying to me a few days earlier, "is to be stronger than she is, because after spending a day with Sophie I have the impression that I don't exist any more." By becoming her "thing" Bernadette entered Sophie's world to such an extent that she lost the recognition points of her own identity. Bernadette no longer knew where she had left Sophie. She no longer knew who she was.

Drawn into a game with Sophie, Bernadette became Sophie. But from that time on, the child had no further interest in her. "I want another Bernadette to play with me. Bernadette is all worn out. I want another one."

Catherine was then engaged by the family. She had completed her studies and had had previous experience in looking after mentally retarded children. Soon after she took over, she tried to tell me about her difficulties. "The educator before me must have been tough; I am so scared that I can't sleep at night. I keep dreaming that Sophie kills herself. Her parents bring a court case against me and you blame me. I am afraid of making mistakes. Sophie's left her mark on me. My worrying upsets her and turns her into a demon."

"Catherine's no good to play with," the child said to me.

"Why?"

"Because she's a Catherine without being Catherine, she doesn't know her way."

The girl fell prey to unmanageable tension and lost all sense of direction with Sophie. Sophie became her guide "for better or for worse. . . ." One day, she left the educator and bathed naked in the fountain of the Tuileries.

The contest lasted eight days. Catherine declared herself beaten. "If I went on, I'd go nuts myself."

Jeanne took over. She was a solid girl with all the marks of a well-balanced personality. She had no intellectual curiosity, but she instinctively adopted the right attitude. She perceived clearly that it was her own fear that induced uncontrollable reactions in the child. "It's a battle in which we square off against each other. It needs two to become panic-stricken." Sophie did, in fact, need to be protected against her aggressive drives. The adult's fear increased her own terror and exposed her to danger.

After a year of analytic treatment, the child no longer seemed demented, but she had not yet emerged from her psychosis. She went to school and was relatively easy to live with. The epileptic fits almost ceased, but encopresis continued. "I've got Sophie's measure," Jeanne told me. "When she gets aggressive, I know how to help her. But I still can't believe it; it's so amazing how stable she is now compared to what she was."

Three days after this, Jeanne shut the child in her bedroom and ran out of the house. Fortunately, the mother came home in time to release the child who was by then beside herself and had wrecked everything in the room that could be destroyed. When I saw Jeanne, she was still in a frenzy of anxiety and deaf to all reproaches. "I want to lie down in Sophie's bed," she said between sobs. Sophie's mother fetched her from my house, and at my request took her to a doctor friend who prescribed rest and tranquilizers.

Four days later, I saw Jeanne again. "I don't know what hit me. I got up to monkey tricks like Sophie."

Then her jealousy about Sophie's "illness" came out, in reference to her own relationship with a psychopathic sister. "Her mother gets on my nerves. Only Sophie matters to her. I don't count. When I ran off, I wanted to get at you through Sophie. I was angry because you didn't understand that I needed psychoanalysis, too."

These observations make it clear that when one undertakes the treatment of a psychotic child, one must listen not only to the parents' complaints but also to the claims of the person who temporarily plays the part of substitute mother, for she bears the full weight of the child's murderous anxiety.

In these three instances, each educator put up a defense against anxiety according to what was at work in her own structure. While Catherine refused to take part in the game, Bernadette entered into it by suppressing all resistance within herself until she became Sophie's thing. In a sort of psychodrama, Sophie played out with Bernadette the kind of relationship that existed between herself and her mother, but the parts were switched around—Sophie was the mother and Bernadette the plaything destined to fulfill her, until the time came when Sophie rejected her as scrap. Bernadette, identified as Sophie's "bad object," got up to monkey tricks (to use the child's terminology), and took to *flight*. The child's drama left no apparent imprint on Jeanne until the "crack-up," when she also revealed a form of identification with the child's symptom (flight). Bernadette and Jeanne became annoyed with the child's mother (they were jealous and claimed the right to be ill themselves). In terms of their relationship with me, it was quite clear that a sudden desire erupted for vengeance on what constituted the object of my desire (Sophie). In the transference to me, the reaction found in the mothers of seriously disturbed children was reproduced: I was confronted with a choice of being able to cure Sophie only at the cost of accepting the death of the adult. "If Sophie gets well, what is going to become of me?" was the question that arose at a certain juncture—thus referring the educator back to her own lack that had been temporarily filled by the child's "illness." The child's progress challenged the adult's relation to her own fundamental problem (relation to death, phallus, etc.). The adult takes part in the cure of a psychotic child; he appears on stage with him; a drama is played out and leaves an imprint on the adult, in accordance with his own past history.[23]

Now to sum up. The parents are always implicated in some way in the symptom exhibited by the child.[24] This fact must not be overlooked because it touches on the very mainspring of *resistance,* namely, the unconscious wish that "nothing shall change," found sometimes in the pathogenic parent. The child can respond to this by the desire that "nothing shall move," thus making restitution for his destructive fantasies about his mother by perpetuating his symptom. If a new dimension[25] is to be introduced in the conception of the transference situation, it will be by the analyst's listening to what is being played out in the fantasy world of mother *and* child. The analyst works with a number of transferences. It is not always easy for him with his own fantasies to situate himself in a world where he risks becoming the stake of an alternative: life or death for the child, or his parents, which reawakens the deepest, most primordial persecutory anxiety subsisting in him.

The parents' problem differs according to whether psychosis or neurosis is involved. The difference relates essentially to the special problem raised by analyzing a child who appears, owing to the dual situation with the mother, as a "result" only of his efforts and

[23] Léon Grinberg, "Psicopatología de la identificación y contraidentificación proyectivas y de la contrasferencia," *Revista de psicoanálisis,* Vol. XX, No. 2 (April–June, 1963). The work of Léon Grinberg throws light on the part played in the analysis of certain patients by the analyst's identification with internal objects of the patient, in response to the provocation the latter offers. He describes situations in which the patient provokes emotional responses in the analyst (the analyst thus becoming the passive or active object of the analysand's projections). In these different forms of transference, something of the order of lack-in-being is occasionally encountered. The purpose of fantasy is to fill this—and the different forms of identification apparently always have a certain relation to the way in which they operate in the subject's fundamental fantasy.

[24] On a very different level, according to whether it is a case of neurosis, psychosis, or retardation. The technique of treatment depends both on the structure involved and the age of the child. The problem of adolescence is subject to special rules.

[25] As already pointed out by some of Melanie Klein's followers, such as A.-A. Pichon-Rivière (cf. *Revue française de psychanalyse* [January–June, 1952]).

never as a subject in his communication. Inasmuch as this situation does not come about by the act of the child alone, it may be discerned how much the adult might feel himself to be under attack when his child is being treated.[26]

In the analysis of neurotics (Joy and Dottie), we also have to deal with a collective communication voiced in the child's words. The child confronts us with the shadow of his parents even if, in reality, we do not want to be concerned with them. Only the distinctions made by Lacan between desire, demand, and need, together with his concept of the registers of the Imaginary, the Real, and the Symbolic, make it possible to place the transference on a level where the subject can be helped to discern a meaning in what his demands have brought into play.[27] The words we hear can then be treated in the style of a grand dream,[28] since the field of play of the transference is not confined solely to what goes on in the analytic session. Transference does not always appear where the analyst thinks he can perceive it (Dora). The signs of transference may be already in position[29] before analysis begins, and subsequently the analyst only fulfills the task allotted to him in the fundamental fantasy of the subject. In a sense, the match had been played beforehand; in order to change its course, the analyst must be aware of what is directed beyond the Imaginary relationship of the subject to the analyst towards something already inscribed, as it were, in a structure, before he makes his appearance on the scene. It

[26] Analysis dislodges the child from the place he occupies in reality (he *exists*, in the Real, as the mother's fantasy; in this way, he dams up the mother's anxiety or fills her lack). This can only be achieved by helping the pathogenic parent to whom the child is attached.

[27] J. Lacan, in seminar, of June 10, 1959 (unpublished).

[28] Although the analysts of Joy and Dottie understood that transference presupposed an opposition of the Imaginary to the Real, their belief that analysis has a rehabilitating side made it impossible for them to seize upon what was in play in the complaints of the child and the parents. The Symbolic dimension of a situation escaped them.

[29] I have developed this idea in connection with the parents of children under analysis.

is here that the countertransference of the analyst comes into play,[30] in how he blocks the movement of metaphor in himself, provoking *acting-out* (decision) in the subject. This generally means that the analyst has been unsuccessful in safeguarding in the interplay of the transference the Symbolic dimension essential to the continuation of treatment.[31]

Freud's discovery[32] in 1897 was the connection between transference and resistance, conceived as an obstacle in the subject's words to the admission of an unconscious wish. In "Little Hans," Freud brought out the complexity of the transference problem in child analysis, by highlighting how the probing of Hans (his position in relation to knowledge, to sex) had to get through not only his own resistance but also that of his parents and of Freud himself. Hans's communication always stayed on a level that the adult found acceptable. His "illness" occupied a very specific place in the fantasy world of the parents (and of the analyst) so that it became the meeting point for the adults themselves (for the father and Freud). What saved Hans was the fact that beyond an Imaginary relationship between the father and Freud, in which Hans had his place as "ill" and as "child," there could be heard, like an oracle, the word of Freud, situating him in a line of descent, in accordance with an established order. It was then that a message could reach the child from the locus of a symbolic Father, enabling him to situate him-

---

[30] O. Mannoni, "Rêve et transfert," *La Psychanalyse,* Vol. VIII (1963).

[31] Either because he mistakes a fantasy for a real danger (Dottie), or because he does not understand what is in play in the parent, thereby provoking in reality the breaking off of treatment by being unable to give a meaning in words to the resistance he is encountering.

[32] Freud called Fliess his "alter ego," and his letters to him were not meant for the public eye. This Imaginary companion was always present in Freud's writings; he was both help and hindrance in Freud's work, the necessary witness, always being discussed, of Freud's psychoanalysis of himself—until the latter produced the theory that the obstacle did not lie so much in the real Other as in himself. "Something from the profoundest depths of my own neurosis has ranged itself against an advance in the understanding of the neuroses and *you have somehow been involved in it*. The impossibility of writing down that which affects me seems to me designed to hinder our communications." Letter 66, of July 7, 1897.

self as subject of a desire outside the game of trickery that had been going on with the complicity of the adults. In Freud's analyses, the subject's position on the problem of desire arises from an anxiety situation in transference. Analysts (particularly of the American school) have tended to reduce the concept of transference to a form of behavior repeated by the subject with an analyst who is taking over in reality as father figure. Freud made it clear how fantasy constructions affect the subject on the Imaginary plane. In this fantasy, as in the symptom, the analyst has his place, but defining it is no simple matter, as the present study has repeatedly shown. Classical references to ego distortions and to reality leave out of the dialectical game the place to which the analyst must succeed in directing himself, if he wants to help the patient both to make his words start flowing again, and to situate himself in relation to recognition points other than those derived from the overconfident judgment of the doctor. Analytic experience is not intersubjective. The subject is called upon to orient himself in relation to his desire[33]—in the dimension of the Other's desire. The merit of the Kleinian school is that it always talks in terms of anxiety *situations* and depressive persecutory *positions* (and not of stages); this dynamic concept of analytic experience leaves the way open to what can be articulated in terms of signifiers in Melanie Klein's technique. The axis around which she makes all analytic experience with children revolve is the phallus, conceived (as Lacan was to say later) as "signifier of desire, in that it is desire for the desire of the Other."

In raising analytic experience to this level, we can assume a different attitude towards the controversy about transference in child analysis. It is not a matter of finding out whether or not the child can transfer his feelings about the parents with whom he continues to live to the analyst (that would reduce transference to a purely affective experience), but one of succeeding in removing the child from the game of trickery he is playing with the complicity of

[33] It is the place of desire that Lacan causes to arise—beyond object relationships.

his parents. This can be achieved only if we understand that the communications that take place are a collective utterance—transference is an experience involving the analyst, the child, and the parents. The child is not an entity in himself. We approach him, first of all, through the representation the adult has of him (What is a child? What is a "sick" child?). Any challenge to the child has very definite repercussions for the parents, and we can neglect it only at our own peril. We have seen the extent of the Imaginary relationship the parent establishes with the analyst during the treatment of psychotic children. Through this Imaginary relationship, the mother becomes capable of reinvesting herself as mother of a child (recognized by a third person as distinct from herself), and can subsequently allow another phase to begin, in which the child proceeds to participate on his own in the psychoanalytic adventure as subject of a desire. The burden of a massive transference by the mother (made up of total trust and absolute mistrust) on the analyst is a very severe challenge to him. Depending on what prematurely anxiety-producing elements within him are exposed, the situation may provoke persecutory or depressive reactions; only at this cost can he undertake treatment successfully.

CHAPTER III

THE PSYCHOTHERAPY
OF PSYCHOSES

In 1896,[1] Kraepelin described *dementia praecox* as a nosological entity. He regarded the marked deterioration of the intellectual faculties in this illness as irreversible.[2] Fifteen years later, E. Bleuler questioned the validity of the entire classical nosology. Not only was the process of schizophrenic deterioration unproven in his opinion, but he was convinced that the patient was making a fool of his doctor, and he illustrated this thesis by numerous clinical examples.[3] Continuing his father's work, M. Bleuler proposed in 1953 that only severe mental illnesses of organic origin ought to be regarded as incurable. His position did not clarify the matter because it was not found possible to reach agreement on the concept of organicity, and many controversies arose around the scientific verification of the organic hypothesis.[4] The orientation of psychoanalysts working with child psychoses remains generally descrip-

[1] E. Kraepelin, *Psychiatrie* (Leipzig, Barth, 1896).

[2] Cf. P. M. Faergeman's study in *Psychogenic Psychoses* (London, Butterworth, 1963).

[3] E. Bleuler, *Dementia Praecox, oder Gruppe der Schizophrenien* (Leipzig and Vienna, Deuticke, 1911).

[4] M. Bleuler, "Eugen Bleuler's Conception of Schizophrenia: An Historical Sketch," *Bulletin of the Isaac Ray Medical Library,* 1953. The classical attitude crystallized round the work of Lutz (Zurich), which appeared in 1937. He distinguished delirious organic schizophrenia from authentic infantile schizophrenia.

tive in essence, except for the Kleinian school. In effect, this study is closely akin in its form to classical psychiatric research.[5]

The European school of psychiatry is concentrating first and foremost on delimiting the boundaries of schizophrenia and its basic research bears on diagnosis, whereas the English and American schools are much more influenced by the contribution of psychoanalysis. The latter are being reproached for unduly extending the definition of schizophrenia so that they tend to find it everywhere. Basing himself on Lacan's findings concerning the "mirror-stage," Lang proposed in 1958 [6] a working hypothesis that took into consideration a dynamic dimension generally disregarded in diagnosis, even by analysts who are nevertheless anxious not to base psychiatric clinical work with children on a static symptomatology. In their attempts to account for the psychotic condition they tend to superimpose a naturalistic description (tinged with psychoanalysis) on the old psychiatric description. The place of the subject remains unoccupied in such classifications.

R. D. Laing[7] made a special study of the problem. He stresses a

[5] R. Diatkine and C. Stein, "Les Psychoses de l'enfance," *Évolution psychiatrique* (April, 1958). The authors distinguish three clinical forms: (1) The psychotic organizations of childhood, characterized by a massive disturbance of development; (2) Prepsychotic or preneurotic states, which are regarded as "dysharmonious" developments that may endanger the whole development of the subject; (3) Schizophrenia precociously constituted as *dementia praecox*. The position of these authors is similar to that of Heuyer whose conceptions, in turn, are very close to those of Lutz.

[6] J.-L. Lang, "L'Abord psychanalytique des psychoses chez l'enfant," *La Psychanalyse*, Vol. IV (1958). Lang questions the validity of explanations that attempt to pinpoint schizophrenia. Could we not, he asks, conceive of the *paranoic structure* as corresponding exactly to the alienating nature of the mirror-phase, and of the *schizophrenic structure* as characterizing a permanent conflict between a tyrannical ego and an I *in posse?* According to Lang, the *cyclophrenic structure* represents a later stage of the conflict when the *I* periodically falls back towards an alienating ego under pressure from an emerging superego, thus resolving the neurotic's anxiety conflict to his disadvantage. Lang wonders whether psychopathic imbalance might not be the result of deformations of the Imaginary ego just as the *I* is attempting to establish itself. In this work, the author takes analysts to task for reducing their technique to a form of educational psychology.

[7] R. D. Laing and A. Esterson, *Sanity, Madness and the Family* (London, Tavistock, 1964). Interviews with the Abbott family (the daughter had spent ten years in the hospital for paranoid schizophrenia) provided the following material: "The

fact now generally admitted, namely, that there is no more controversial question in medicine than the diagnosis of schizophrenia. Psychiatry, he tells us, has been particularly concerned with behavior regarded by society as abnormal; such behavior has been categorized into symptoms and signs of supposedly pathological syndromes or illnesses, but no objective criteria for the diagnosis of schizophrenia have been discovered. Every conceivable view is held by the various authorities. There are no pathological anatomical findings post mortem, nor are there organic structural changes noted in the course of the "illness." Laing adds that schizophrenia runs in families, but observes no evident genetic law and occurs in every constitutional type.

Laing then examines what he calls the *career* of a patient diagnosed as schizophrenic. He records different types of communication—those of the patient, of the patient's parents, and of the patient with each parent. Without comment, he provides a sort of summary for each case, in which the patient's point of view about his "illness" is set out side by side with the parents'. Thus we are reading a series of monographs.

In one of these (the Abbotts), the place of the daughter in the fundamental fantasy of the mother is revealed in a particularly striking fashion. The daughter formed part of the mother's organs, in the latter's fantasy and, imagining that the daughter might eventually attain the state of being the subject with desire, the mother prayed to God that her daughter remain forever in the hospital. An interview with the daughter's doctor was deemed unnecessary by the mother because it was obvious that she could not get better. "Society is not meant for her." Laing demonstrates by means of

---

young woman said that blackness came over her when she was eight. This was denied by the parents; they alone were in a position to know, they told us, that her memory was at fault. They alone knew what she was feeling and what she was thinking. They alone knew whether she masturbated or not. They alone knew if she had sexual thoughts concerning her parents. When the daughter asked them whether they could read her mind, they replied in the affirmative. 'There is nothing for her to understand,' said the mother, 'her illness made her do it. If she can't remember, she tries to imagine what happened.' " The family thus reflects the position of classical psychiatry: there is no room in it for a subject.

many clinical examples how catatonic and paranoid symptoms, auditory hallucinations, impoverishment of affect, and autistic withdrawal appeared as echoes of the parents' communication. The panic registered by the parents was not so much the effect of their child's "illness" as of the problems raised by a prospective cure. Her mother anxiously questioned her daughter at regular intervals to make sure that she was still "ill." The daughter bore the hallucinatory imprint of words (those of her mother or of both parents). Words from all sides kept her compressed in a vise, beset her, wounded her, harassed her. All outlets were blocked—her madness had to continue. "My daughter can't recover her memory," the mother said, "her illness makes her need us." Thus everything was organized in the family's communication in order that the subject have no desire of her own.

What has been heard in the family determines the delusional, hallucinated, and autistic words of a child and reinforces the primordial severity of a superego which has become terrifying. The child (as Melanie Klein has shown) feels himself exposed at a very tender age to the threat of interior aggression; projected onto the exterior it unveils for him a surrounding world which he perceives as dangerous on the fantasy plane. This situation of aggressive projection occurs (according to the Kleinian school) in all normal children at the culmination of the Oedipus stage; the superego is supposed to be the result of introjecting a terrifying parental figure. But, if the parent proves to be in fact "threatening" in reality, the normal building-up of a superego does not take place and the child is delivered over to the fantastic effects of his own projections in a situation of pure mirror-aggressiveness. All conflicts are then lived in terms of the alternative of suicide or murder. At the same time, the child feels himself to be in danger, because he has not acquired an image of himself as a unified body; the absence of identification between his ego and the mirror-ego drives him to flee from his own body[8] and to remain constantly alienated in some part of it

[8] Cf. Piera Aulagnier, "Remarques sur la structure psychotique," *La Psychanalyse*, Vol. VIII (1963).

(mouth, anus). Only at this price can he maintain himself in his mother's desire and situate himself in the adult's dialectics. These are the baselines for a subsequent development of schizophrenia.

Every time that Christiane (aged six) showed a desire for autonomy, her mother intervened on the Real plane to make it forever impossible to sever the ties between them. She induced her daughter's somatic complaint by enemas and medicines that she administered without the doctor's knowledge. She examined her stools and watched over her diet. The child could not escape, for in escaping she would have to lose her mother. On the level of the Real, the mother manifested herself only in anal or oral aggressions—this was where her gift of love was situated. Christiane alternately rejected her mother and then became alienated from herself again in order to find her. She made herself not only a mouth to be fed and an anus to be filled, but she even lost herself as subject in educational games. With precise gestures, she would tap the balloon into the basket, or work out the most complicated puzzles, but her activity was never mediated by a human image—so that a ball, or, indeed, any toy, could never serve as a medium of exchange between herself and the other. There was no other; it was she herself in her body who was the medium of exchange and who lost herself in the object. Christiane knew her body (she could enumerate all its parts), but this intellectual knowledge was divorced from any integration with an accurate physical awareness. She lacked spatial or sensory knowledge of her body. She bumped into pieces of furniture, fell over every obstacle. "I have to be there," said the mother, "for Christiane to find her feet. Look where you're going—here's a hole, there's a wall, and that's the door there." Caught in the net of her mother's look, Christiane was the little ball that remained suspended in mid-air, the hole that opened and shut. She revealed the extent to which she was divided into bits and pieces by the way her words were fragmented. She stammered out every word with terrible difficulty; only her mother understood her inarticulate speech.

In effect, the mother was not prepared to give her daughter to anyone. Analysis became a suspect enterprise the moment it seemed likely to touch on her personal positions. Despite an outward appearance of extreme fragility, she was a woman who had things and people firmly under her thumb. She used doctors as alibis. She gave them up as soon as they expressed a wish that ran counter to her own. She had no communication with her daughter beyond lessons and physical attentions. She took care to assume the conduct of the treatment, undoing by words what it had been possible to build up in a session. Every time the child might have established a link, the mother interposed to keep her aware of the possibility of a break.

Christiane's mother had fulfilled the desire of a paranoid father by continuing with her studies against her own wish—and she then cancelled out this faithfulness to her father's wish by making no use in her life of the possibilities that her qualifications offered her. She became a housewife, but in the care she lavished on her daughter she endeavored to prove the futility of all effort. She who had witnessed her father's madness now witnessed her daughter's, and she looked for his stigmata (allergic rashes) on the child's body. Christiane was thus destined to remain in a particular place. Any improvement brought on depression in her mother.

In touching on Christiane's psychosis, one was touching on the place occupied by the mother, as persecutory object, in her own father's delusions. She reduced her child to being her sexual object in order to re-create with her a form of Oedipal link.

During the child's treatment, it was from the mother that the crises arose, and it was in her words that resistance could be read. The child bore witness by her reserve to the effect on her of her mother's hostility towards me. At the outset of treatment, the mother had defined its limits to me: "I shall stay with Dr. X so long as I can't find anyone better. I have no more faith in him than in the others." There was hardly room for belief in my words. Some dramatic incidents involving the mother had occurred in the course of treatment before the child started to participate on her own. Precisely at that juncture, the mother suspended it. Christiane, aware of the new drama being played around her, remained torn between a tyrannical *ego* (which referred her to her mother's words and the latter's failure to recognize), and an *I* which could not emerge for lack of a third who could be the guarantor of a *law of language* (and protect her from the murderous word which cancelled out the meaning of words).

According to Kleinian theories, all human beings pass through psychotic stages[9] during childhood. The role of the real mother is to modify the baby's fantasy life by countering its Imaginary terrors with a reassuring presence which translates into meaningful speech. From birth, the baby experiences an intense form of anxiety resulting from separation from the mother. It remains sensitized to her presence and absence, which it lives as fusion and separation. Later tests, such as weaning, are approached with the same process of recurrence,[10] which implies for the subject the overcoming of his primal death tendency. A failure at this level is the seedbed from which certain psychotic difficulties develop—difficulties that generally occur before the age of seven months. Something of cardinal importance is enacted in what Lacan calls the "mirror-stage" (six months). The test of separation has already brought into play the Imaginary link between the subject and the Other. At a later stage, the child will assume his image (as a totality), and the image of his counterpart as being different from his own. Self-knowledge dates from the time when he recognizes his own image. The jubilant moment he experiences marks a victory over the confrontation in the mirror, which in a psychotic brings about self-destruction, or the destruction or negation of the Other. The baby acquires this knowledge of himself as a revelation through the mediating image of his mother or her substitute, and when such image is lacking,

[9] Schizo-paranoid position during the first three months of life. Depressive position during a later phase.

[10] Cf. J. Lacan, "La Famille," in *La Vie mentale,* Vol. VIII of the *Encyclopédie française* (Paris, Société de Gestion de l'Encyclopédie Française, 1938).

the child cannot pass the test and takes refuge in destruction. The encounter with his image through that of the other leads on to the knowledge of himself and other people, by means of a crisis of identificatory jealousy in which the fate of reality is at stake. The subject, forced into the choice, must decide either to come to terms with the other or to destroy him. In psychotics, destruction takes the place of any possibility of human sympathy.

Leon, caught in the net of his parents' murderous words, felt himself to be in danger under their eyes, as if he were risking death by being seen.[11] Love lived in terms of oral aggression engendered a terror of being devoured. While Leon was making progress in treatment, the analyst had to contend with the murderous words of the mother in periods of crisis: "If only he could die of it," she would say in front of her son. Petrified, trapped, the child refused to speak lest his words prove equally dangerous.

Leon's progress under treatment occurred through a development in the parents' communication, in that they told me what the child himself did not say, thus allowing him to be born as a phallic plus-value.[12] When the words around him radically changed, the child entered the treatment as subject in his symptom; the day it was possible to tackle with Leon the fact that he had been playing at being mad marked a decisive turning-point. The effects were shown in an awareness of his own body; he rapidly acquired the habit of cleanliness, and began urinating like a boy, which he had previously refused to do standing up. He learned to swim, excelled in games involving physical dexterity, and adjusted to a kindergarten class.

His relationship with his parents remained difficult; he accepted

[11] The child could not bear to see himself in the mirror, since the meaning of the image of himself as seen by another referred him to the adults' death-wishes.

[12] *Phallic plus-value:* The real child symbolizes the phallus for the mother. As he develops, the child must take over the phallus on his own, but this is only possible after he has achieved a mirror-image of himself. The mother must accept herself as the locus of lack, to enable the child to realize himself independently of her, and become the mother's phallic plus-value and not her phallus.

the triangular situation only if they kept talking about him. His "illness" was thus eroticized and occupied a certain place in the adults' discourse. The son's cure plunged the father into a series of depressive attacks, for it prevented the development of a purely homosexual relationship. (The parents had established a modus vivendi—the mother busied herself with the daughter, the father with the son, and the sex life of the parents had virtually ceased.)

The child's development had to be accomplished therefore by means of challenging the parents and changing a situation in which he could not situate himself as the son of so-and-so. He was Daddy's wife and Mummy's safety valve. The child's fixation on his psychotic defenses (related to the alienating side of the mirror-stage) was maintained by his father who was himself in difficulties with his Oedipal problem.

The transition from the narcissistic phase to the Oedipal phase is a decisive one—the Oedipal phase introduces a new structure through the part played by Oedipal identification. We re-enter the domain of the phallus and the Name of the Father; in the relationship of the subject to the Other, the foreclosure of one of these terms is characteristic of psychosis. Such foreclosure falsifies the entire relationship of the subject to reality[13] by causing the loss of either his Imaginary or his Symbolic function. We know that reality can be experienced only if these two correlating functions are maintained intact, and failure in the Imaginary or the Symbolic register is thus the hallmark of the psychotic phenomenon. A person suffering from delusions[14] makes use of language to demonstrate his own exclusion as subject. The schizophrenic, on the other hand, lives in a world where the Symbolic has taken over the place of the Real, but without any link to the Imaginary.

---

[13] The study of S. Leclaire in *Évolution psychiatrique* (April, 1958), "A la recherche d'une psychothérapie des psychoses," should be consulted in this connection. Based on the works of Lacan, it endeavors to pinpoint what is in play in the psychotic phenomenon. A work on theory, it opens up a clinical approach in the treatment of psychoses.

[14] A person suffering from delusions respects the laws of language. A schizophrenic's speech is disordered.

Lucien (fourteen years old) spoke in a manner that was striking for its musical intonations. Standing in front of me, with a fixed look, he pumped words out jerkily, in a high-pitched voice; occasionally, there was a pause on a solemn note, an inaudible murmur, then he would start again, like a phonograph record:[15] "It isn't poisonous? I don't want to be dead, I don't want to be dead, I shall not be dead. *Thursday*. Mr. Freddy is dead, but that doesn't count. He was greedy. He ate three whole chickens and he didn't listen to the doctor. I shall never be dead, I shall never be old, *because I don't want to*. I like going to Juvisy, it's a well-ventilated establishment where you get things to eat; it isn't a school, even if it is a school, because it hasn't got school written on it, *but I want to leave*. It's poisonous, I don't want to be dead, I shall never be dead. *I don't want to be touched*. Are you a lady? You ought to know, I don't know anything, you are the one who knows. I say that to everyone when I talk to find out." Indifferent, pathetic, Lucien suddenly shut his eyes and started to sway. When he touched his interlocutor, he annulled it immediately by taking refuge in a sort of hallucination, curled up in the fetal position, making sucking motions.

The manner of his speech, fading in and out, indicated Lucien's presence and his fall. A remark from the analyst touching on his persecutory anxiety started him up again, the words revolving in a vacuum. (Intense panic was followed by sleep.) "It isn't poisonous. Show me how to say it. Show me how to speak. Show me how to say it. I don't know how to speak. *I don't know at all. I don't know anything. I'm tired. You're the one who knows.*" Inhabited by the Other's words, crammed, constrained, trapped from his earliest years by the constant presence of an adult who "would not let him go," Lucien at times cut himself off from the world. It was likely that he was hallucinating a breast, indeed that he was the hallucinated breast. Thumb in his mouth he dreamed, rocking to and fro, and then, hands on his knees, he curled up, still rocking, as the thumb-sucking gave way to sucking motions of his lips. What exactly was Lucien hallucinating? Was it his mother's breast? The

[15] Italicized words were uttered on a solemn note.

expression and set of the boy's face appeared to be seeking something to complete it, to fill the cavity of the mouth. He conveyed what he was looking for in a complaint: "Mummy, blanket, nice and warm." Whining and sucking motions alternated. Lucien himself fixed the limits of the dream within which he wished to shut himself, not as the subject accepting severance from his mother's body, but identifying with a part of her body, forming a whole out of that part, thereby denying a reality from which he was excluded as subject. He inscribed himself in this reality as a cavity, achieving completeness within himself.

In this hallucinatory activity, Lucien achieved his negation as subject, refusing reality if it had to be severed from his own body. For Lucien, this breast not only did not belong to an Other but evoked nothing in the region beyond the Other. Thus, by means of the twofold negation[16] he could retain the basically satisfying object. He refused to run the risk of being unsatisfied, a risk linked to the recognition that the breast belonged to the Other and was consequently subject to withdrawal. Lucien established his enclosed space and achieved within himself the negation of the reality of his own existence—the existence of a being calling for help from an emptiness and from a lack of being.

The manner in which the psychotic cuts himself off, not only from any relationship with the Other but also from any relationship with his own body, was studied by Freud in *Mourning and Melancholia*. The premature rejection of a beloved being in reality can be transformed, he tells us, into a loss of ego which serves as a prelude to entering a psychotic state. He gives us clinical examples of subjects suppressing or injuring themselves in identifying with a beloved object they had rejected. These ideas provided the basis for the Kleinian theories about child psychoses. However, it was Karl Abraham who first conceived the idea that the existence of a depressive situation in children might serve as a model for adult mel-

16 Insofar as he was not severed from his mother's body and that reality was not severed from his own body.

ancholia. His hypothesis was confirmed by Melanie Klein, then at the beginning of her career, when she undertook the psychoanalysis of a three-year-old child.

We have seen that the analytic situation can readily be perceived as dangerous, in that it is lived by the subject in terms of an alternative (either he injures himself or he attacks the object he fears outside himself). When the analyst seeks to introduce himself by his words into the world of an alienated child, he meets with a wish for complete exclusion, even a murder wish. Although apparently deaf to the adult's words, the psychotic's play nevertheless bears witness to the fact that something has been understood. The interpretation of aggression in relation to a very clearly defined anxiety situation (linked to the child's position in regard to his parents) makes it possible to continue treatment, even if it is marked by frequent periods of persecutory or depressive tension. The analyst's use of the right word (which touches on the very source of the subject's sadism[17]) unblocks a flow of communication which tends continually to shut down again in a closed circuit. But this work with the child always awakens a form of anxiety in the analyst; sometimes, he unconsciously protects himself by trying to leave the actual scene of analysis.

The idea of traumatism as the explanation of certain morbid processes was introduced by Freud, but it was subsequently perceived that the future effects of a painful event for the subject were linked to the way in which the event was dealt with in the adults' words. The adult's words leave a greater imprint on the child than the event itself. Often, it is only after considerable time has gone by following the real incident that one can succeed in situating that element which has been selected as its traumatic effect. The fate of the psychotic hinges less on a real perturbing event than on the way the subject has been excluded by one parent or the other from the possibility of entering a triangular structure. This is what dooms him to be arrested at the stage of a partial object, without ever

---

[17] That is, touches on the severity of the superego.

assuming an identity of his own. It is instructive to hear a pyschotic child's speech in conjunction with that of the pathogenic parent; the analyst discerns the place occupied by the child in the parent's fantasy, a place that precludes his own accession to the state of sexualized subject. The parent's word can remain such that it forever blocks the child's accession to his own word.

The Martin family had three children, aged ten, eight, and five. The eldest, Denis, appeared to be profoundly feeble-minded, his body petrified in panic. The daughter, Veronique, was psychotic. The youngest child was entering a condition of anorexia. The parents were overwhelmed and appealed to the authorities to take charge of the two older children. The mother was a frequent inmate of mental hospitals, and the father was often away traveling, absorbed in his work; he also had bouts of depression. Let us listen to them at random, as they talked during sessions.

Father: "Denis was always sick till he was six years old—it cleared up when he was boarded out. His sister copies whatever her brother does. I don't see any way out. His mother is almost off her head. We shall have to have one of them put away. My wife has been hopelessly impaired. When Denis was seven, his mother was pregnant and depressed. Denis ran around in the streets. We gave his sister the chance. As for the oldest one, we just said 'too bad.' I have accepted my oldest as being as good as dead. I have become resigned to it while he's still alive."

Denis: "Where's Daddy? Where's Mummy? Are they going to let me fall?"

Mother: "Denis is O.K., he's manageable. Veronique is hopeless. I brought her up like an animal, because her brother was always sick. I was always having rows with my husband. Veronique went without everything. Denis was stuffed to his ears. She lived in an abnormal atmosphere. Denis was scared of everything. The boy was the one I loved, I never looked at the girl. I kept the two children isolated, I was ashamed of them."

Denis: "They're not going to eat me? What happens if I draw?"

Mother: "Veronique is too much under Denis' influence. She's withdrawn from the world. Sometimes she's normal, sometimes she gets miserable—she doesn't get on with her father. I bully Denis and my husband bullies her. I'm afraid for the youngest."

Veronique: "I'm fed up with Denis. I cry and they give me something to eat. How do you hold a doll? Can I draw? What happens if I draw?"

Mother: "The two children look at each other as if they could kill each other."

Denis and Veronique lived a murder fascination in mirror-image. Each had the feeling that he could succeed in living only at the cost of the other's death. Each lived in total panic at the physical level. All desire was forbidden. All wishes brought with them the danger of death. The children did not even look human. They were little wild beasts, trapped and rooted to the ground by ungovernable fear. The parents were totally deficient. The words surrounding the children precluded the possibility of their ever being born to a desire of their own. Their persecutory anxiety was the response to the depressive anxiety of their parents. The words of the children reflected the words of the adults.

Here is another example. Adrien had been mute since the age of three when he had been separated from his mother for the fifth time; she had been sent to the hospital on several occasions, each time urgently, for fits of depression. "For three months they were at him, all the time trying to get him to talk. But it wasn't any good. Since the time he was boarded out, it's been catastrophic. If they hadn't brought him back, he'd have died of it." The parents had lived for five years in a single room without running water. The day they were given decent accommodations, the mother had another attack of depression. Bearing the imprint of a childhood she described as a "martyrdom," the woman started feeling guilty and anxious as soon as things seemed to be going a little better. She needed witnesses to her personal drama. She tried to stay alienated in the depths of a fantasy; she did not want the meaning revealed to her. "A childhood like that sticks to you forever. It was like being dead, nothing could be worse than what I've lived through." All the children in the family were more or less seriously disturbed. "Adrien hugs me and I scream at him for it, he torments me so. And the sicker I feel, the naughtier Corine is." The home was like hell itself. Each child was the veritable destroyer of the other. The mother lived in dread of being raped. If aggression was not expressed in the external world, it was enacted by the children. In words and deeds, they conveyed the effects of their mother's terror on them. "I was shoved around," said the mother, "from one place to another. My mother couldn't stand the sight of me. I didn't understand the dreadful things she used to say to me. I wouldn't want my children to go through what I went through. I ran away when I was eleven. I cut myself off from my family for good." She did not know how to be a mother. "I haven't learned how," she said. The children were well looked after and the house was sparkling clean, but she had no words to give. "I haven't learned how to speak." When she did let out words, they simply wreaked havoc. Adrien's muteness bore witness to what had remained uncommunicable in the mother. His appointed task was to screen what the mother sought to hide from herself. This was akin to the drama of incest (lived either in reality or on the Imaginary plane; it was difficult to disentangle fact from fiction in the accusations she made). In her words, she explained in various forms that her own children and her children's children were forever accursed, and that no one would ever succeed in atoning for the crime she accused herself of—that of having been desired, as a child, by her mother's man. "From the time I was quite small, I was like his wife to him. I went along with it. Then when I was eleven I ran away, and a little while later my father died. I caused his death." She lived in fear of a vengeance. The domestic hell was her guarantee of her right to live. The serious disorders of the children, known to all the neighbors, took the place of a crime that had to remain forever hidden.

We have seen earlier in the case of Emile how he occupied a place of being dead in his mother's fantasy and how he was linked to the Oedipal history of the mother who was fixated on her father who had committed suicide. This psychotic, organically deficient child (encephalopathy and epilepsy) made rapid progress which corresponded to a radical change in the mother's words. When he was no longer held in a net of murderous fantasies, he was able to accede to words ("pretty Mummy"), eat by himself, become neat, and acquire a certain degree of motor autonomy. He took over the use of his penis and of his body as soon as he entered a triangular situation; he had to confront, through the father, the anthropophagic taboo and the taboo against incest. The child could be born to life (that is to say, face castration) as soon as the mother said, "I'd rather have a son who leads a dog's life than a son who stays an idiot." From the moment the mother accepted the child's castration (and no longer talked of its killing her) the child was able to begin to live with what he lacked.

As soon as Sophie's mother no longer responded by a sort of fusion to her daughter's epileptic fits, Sophie was able to enter as the subject of desire, and not as a partial object, into the castration dialectics. Up to then, Sophie had been playing—through her encopresis, her fits, her bouts of temperature—a sort of fetishistic game designed to screen her severance from her mother's body. What came out in Sophie's analysis was the series of masquerades she used against anxiety, as well as the different forms of repudiation that served to mask the existence of castration. Sophie was trying to escape in her masquerades from the identification to which the desire of the Other was referring her, and she thus remained stuck on a seesaw, caught in a twofold negation—one touching on the object of desire (which she could not conceive of losing), and the other touching on the object of demand (she was trying to possess the partial object at the risk of denying the desire of the Other). In her paralyzing questions, "Do I want to come?

Don't I want to come?" Sophie was expressing a splitting on the identification level and revealing in this fashion her desire to keep everything and lose nothing. She could maintain this desire only by denying reality; she substituted for it obedience to the pleasure principle alone.

The diagnosis before she started treatment had been a congenital encephalopathy, its etiology being linked, it was thought, to a prenatal infection. When she was five, the various doctors who had been consulted had no doubts about either the seriousness of the encephalopathy or the organic nature of the clinical signs of convulsions. In the opinion of some specialists, the only possible diagnosis was insanity. From her birth, the mother had been haunted by the idea that Sophie might die. The child was suffering from sobbing spasms, epileptic fits, and severe intestinal infections, all causing relatively long stays in the hospital. From her infancy on, Sophie had been looked after by a number of people; she was appealing to her mother through her illnesses. During her long absences, the mother would entrust the child to her own mother, who never ceased to mourn her daughter's marriage. It was only after Sophie started analysis that her mother was able to invest in the child *as mother*. Until then the child had always seemed to her to belong by right to her own mother. From her entry into the world, Sophie had been situated outside any symbolic field, invested as a "leftover" to be given to the grandmother. Very early in the analysis, the mother's hatred for her own mother appeared in the foreground together with the previously unrecognized Oedipal problem. It was precisely from that base (i.e., her renunciation of her father) that the mother's communication with her husband about the child could be re-ordered. She was not a schizophrenic-type mother but a hysteric. She had succeeded in keeping her self-composure by not allowing herself to be marked by anything (not letting herself be "got at" either by grief or love; her relationship with her husband was primarily narcissistic).

What about organicity in Sophie's case? In retrospect, the entire diagnosis, though carefully made in various hospitals, could probably be challenged. If there really had been organic damage, the child could not have changed so quickly as to be educable after eighteen months of treatment. The child indicated the weak point in her mother's armor by her madness and her organic symptoms, while by her hypersexuality she denounced the sexual deficiency of her parents. Sophie took pleasure in the smell of excrement, she was destructive, dirty, screaming, and ugly. She was born to the condition of being a girl during treatment, or rather, she became narcissistic and began to feel capable of risking being a girl in all respects.

In sum, the hypothesis of prenatal injury has been advanced for Sophie, Emile, Christiane, and Leon. An organic factor seemed to be closely associated with the psychogenic disorder. The children in the Martin family looked like inmates of an asylum. In the cases of Leon and Sophie it became possible to discard the hypothesis of organicity and ascribe the disorder solely to the psychogenic factor. As for Christiane, her parents were so committed to believing in a physical cause of her disorder that the psychoanalytic experiment was foredoomed. Emile's encephalopathy was indisputable, yet his improvement under treatment was so great that it demonstrated the part played by a subsequent psychogenic factor, namely, the imprint of a type of maternal anxiety on the level of the child's body. The Martins, like Christiane's parents, did not propose to be challenged through their children's treatment. The former demanded that the children be put away while the latter wanted to keep a controlling hand on the conduct of the treatment, which implied that organicity was to remain unquestioned. The parents of Lucien had been consulting doctors in France and abroad for over ten years, then waited until Lucien reached the age of fourteen before beginning analytic treatment that had been recommended when the child was five. "If somebody had told me that I was condemning my child by interrupting his treatment, I should have carried on with it," the mother exclaimed. Unfortunately, experience with similar cases shows us that nothing of the sort is likely to occur. A favorable prognosis in all these severe cases depends mainly on the parents' manner of communication—the petrified closed-circuit manner which evokes judgment, or the dramatic manner which appeals for help.

The murder wish (or the unconscious desire that the child stay ill) exists openly or under various guises; in both cases, we have seen that there was no room for a subject in the mother's words as heard by the child. When the parents address themselves to the analyst *for* their "sick" child, they are talking indirectly about themselves in speaking about him. We must pay heed to two distinct types of message:

1. What I have called *closed-circuit* communication, encountered particularly with Christiane's mother and also with the parents of Denis and Veronique. It is recited *in the analyst's presence* rather than directed *to the analyst*.

Christiane's mother deplored the disorder from which her daughter suffered; she related a detailed anamnesis flawlessly and rigorously; she produced facts, and her view of things was presented as objective. "That's the exact truth," she said. This truth was in fact an objectivating discourse which left no room for the subject's word and closed the door on its truth. The child's past was re-ordered, not to bring out a meaning but simply to establish it. The mother "held forth" about her child. Her remarks were addressed to herself, and it was she again who held the key to the response. She situated the analyst in the position of conniving with her own lies. There was no room for a third party, Christiane's mother being that third party for herself. We may observe in all such cases that the pathogenic parent constitutes himself as the ego-ideal; any outside intervention may expose him to discomfiture and an aggressive break occurs as a defense mechanism. If the analyst does not intervene, he remains powerless and cannot disengage the child's words from the parental symptom—but if he does intervene, he generally precipitates a decision to break off the treatment.

The words of the parents of Denis and Veronique did not differ much from those of Leon's or Emile's mother, except in one particular. The latter mothers had a message for their child's analyst; the message may be slowly transformed, depending on the recipient, and the possibility of completely altering the initial text is of crucial importance for the chances of developing a cure. The parents of Denis and Veronique had some points in common with Christiane's, namely, that the indictment they voiced was what other people had said about them. "It's domestic hell," the parents seemed to be saying, "how do you expect a child to make out under conditions like this?" The analyst is called as witness to a drama which in itself constitutes a reply that cannot be challenged. If he endorses the parents' words, he keeps up their visits. If he intervenes as a third party, he puts them to flight. The "sick" child is the representative or prop of the parents' disorder, but it is a disorder they want to keep foreclosed. Christiane's parents wanted to keep their "sick" child at home whereas Denis' parents wanted to get rid of him, but the style of the approaches was identical: they could not be challenged. It was impossible to make use of their words in treating the child, because they were situated outside any dialectical movement. A message had first to be released from them, not from the child.

2. In what I have referred to as the *communication of drama,* the analyst is struck by the ruthless nature of the murder wishes expressed by the parents with respect to the child. The anxiety thereby aroused in the analyst may be utilized in treatment, however, in contrast to that produced by the parents in the first group; the analyst participates in the dialectical movement which is being worked out. The mother's response, "This is what I am like," is in fact a question, "What should I become in all this, and can I count on you?" Hate, revolt, refusal, covering up, will in these circumstances have the meaning they assume in all analyses. The drama to which we are referred is not that of the child's "illness" but the parents' drama of existence. As soon as there is a recognition related to

the Oedipal problem of the father or mother, the child is enabled to present himself as subject in his symptom. Previously, his mother has invested him in reality as a fantasy. (The analyst, with the agreement of the parents, has occasion at a certain point in treatment to speak of their Oedipal problem to the child.)

We know that in an adult analysis the birth of a subject in his word is accomplished from the baseline of death. When we are dealing with a child caught in the death-wishes of his parents, it is their words first of all which must be unraveled. To the extent that the parents are blocked on the Symbolic plane, the child feels compelled to remain petrified for them, in the place of one dead though still alive.

In starting to treat a pyschotic child, one is drawn into a drama through the interaction of the parents' words and those of the child. This presupposes that the analyst can succeed in detecting fairly accurately the fashion in which child and parents find themselves stuck in their positions with regard to desire. It is not necessary to analyze the parents, but it is essential to recognize that which in the adults' words has left its imprint on the child at the physical level.

In the conduct of treatment, the clinical approach depends on the therapist's theoretical orientation. Rosenfeld [18] noted that all psychotherapeutic techniques, regardless of theory, score successes in the acute phase of the illness. It is a very different matter in the phase described as one of chronic silence, and a successful outcome depends entirely on how this is handled. The Kleinian school has demonstrated the importance of strict analysis from the acute phase. Whether the analysis is successful depends on an understanding of the psychotic mechanism in transference situations. Here, the analyst's countertransference leads him all too often to abandon classical technique. His own anxiety, facing as he is the aggressive projections of the patient, drives him to find methods of reassur-

[18] H. Rosenfeld, "Notes on the Psychoanalysis of the Superego Conflict in an Acute Schizophrenic Patient" in Melanie Klein *et al.,* eds., *New Directions in Psychoanalysis* (London, Tavistock, 1955; New York, Basic Books, 1956).

ance, but he thereby mishandles everything in the patient's words that touches on abandonment, death, destruction, and condemnation.

Some people regard the psychotic as one seriously traumatized, to whom happiness must be brought in the form of what it was he had missed having.[19] An attempt is made here to substitute various pleasures or even gifts for what the patient did not get, without pausing to consider whether the lack in question was of the order of an object frustration in reality (creating an Imaginary injury[20]), or if the deprivation occurred in the Symbolic order, provoking the child to break with reality. A child's demand can aim at satisfying a need, but beyond the demand for food there is always one for something else,[21] and the object given or refused by the mother is invested by the child as a sign of love. The appeal for love maintains in him an unsatisfied dimension that can never be entirely filled. Thus the child spends his time sending out his demands for signs of love beyond the satisfaction of a need. It is the "something else," as such, that he desires. If the mother cannot endure this lack, this emptiness from which the child makes his appeal, she will stop him from articulating something that lies beyond the demand, beyond the maternal function. The Symbolic outlet will be blocked by the all-powerful presence of the mother intervening in reality on the level of need. If the analyst then takes over from the mother by providing a response in reality, he might make the situation worse and perpetuate the confusion between the register of need and the register of desire; he might thus mask the appearance of a lack of being which the subject had not been able to signify until he started analysis.

In the analytic situation, it is precisely when the psychotic child is bringing something essential into play at the level of *desire* that he

[19] M. A. Séchehaye, *A New Psychotherapy in Schizophrenia,* trans. Grace Rubin-Rabson (New York, Grune & Stratton, 1956).

[20] Developed by J. Lacan in his seminars 1956–7.

[21] Developed by M. Safouan, "Le phallus dans le rapport mère-enfant" (unpublished).

is trying to keep it at the level of *demand,* thereby taking refuge in a deceptive reality. When Sophie began to have an inkling that she was playing at being mad in order to please me, she switched immediately into the register of reality, looking for another mask. She was afraid to appear unveiled before the Other's gaze, as if her entry into the desire of the Other were tantamount to her disappearing as subject. In the analytic situation, Sophie used her body as the stake in a game. She provoked me into worrying by trying to jump out the window, but the interpretation that she was trying to please me by her "illness" made her run to the kitchen with a demand for food. This flight had a direct relationship in reality to an interpretation which was correct as far as it went but was not sufficiently subtle. In it, I emphasized the way in which the child situated herself in relation to my desire as partial object, and thus provoked, for want of adequate verbalization, a sort of acting-out. The interpretation, instead of dealing with the analyst's pleasure, ought to have dealt with the pleasure of the subject, which would have precluded the panic effect caused by the dual situation. As Lacan reminds us, in the analytic situation the third party is always present; it is up to the analyst to proceed in such a way that it emerges. The third party is the judge of the truth that comes out of the words directed at the analyst. In the case of psychoses, the analyst must allow his own desire to be tracked down and unmasked by the subject to allow the third party to intervene. "You are giving yourself pleasure" does not have the same defensive meaning as "You are giving me pleasure." [22] In the first case, I put the stress on one of the terms and leave open for the subject the possibility of an interplay of substitute signifiers. In the second, I unintentionally block this operation and invite the subject to take refuge in a reality that signifies the child's refusal to accept the Symbolic dimension. When Sophie was trying (by attacking me) to maintain herself on the level of a desire, I brought her back to a demand, making it

[22] The correct interpretation could also have been made in the form of the question, "To whom do you want to give pleasure?"

impossible to uncover the meaning. Demands for milk, bananas, or apples always come up in analytic sessions as a response to my own anxiety. Mothering is the outcome of an anxiety situation and I find it hard to endure it, which the child perceives as such. The flight kitchenward—which I have always accepted so that I could grasp its meaning—has occurred with a number of psychotic children. It has always been the reaction to the same type of interpretation, one felt by the subject to be the effect of a dual situation. By polarizing on the analyst instead of on the subject, I caused the disappearance of the Other as locus of truth. What remained was an Imaginary fascination that could find no outlet except in flight and gave the analyst no chance to bring the Symbolic dimension to light. Analytic action takes place on a level other than that of pure relational technique. By lending herself in an ingenuous fashion to the "good mother" game, she (or he) is volunteering to approve the trap which the subject is trying to keep up. But it is the analyst's job to flush the patient out of the trap so that he can emerge from the confusion into which his psychosis has plunged him.[23] What is commonly termed oral or anal regression, and so on, does not seem to be a return to an earlier stage of development, but rather a means employed by the subject to decorate himself and thereby insure that he will be recognized. This is transposed into the mishaps of communication. In Sophie's case, the demand for milk seemed like a flight into reality to avoid interference in her status as one who desires. In the flight, she deceived herself and made a fool of her interlocutor as well.

We must remember the very special place the psychotic occupies in the field of the mother's desire. When the child cannot gain recognition by the Other in his status as subject who desires, he becomes alienated in a part of his body.[24] The child's relationship with his mother remains in a field from which he has no outlet but

[23] Confusion between the Real and the Symbolic registers.

[24] Piera Aulagnier, "Remarques sur la structure psychotique," *La Psychanalyse,* Vol. VIII (1963).

the perpetual renewal of demands, without ever acquiring the right to assume desire. In effect, he enters his mother's dialectics as a partial object. The interdependence between mother and child, the tyranny of the link that joins them, is equally strong on both sides. In his relationship with us, the psychotic makes the Other the object of his introjection (Christiane, Leon, Sophie, Emile), or else he speaks from another locus infinitely remote, and the words he voices are not his own (Lucien). Both ways, the subject has not been severed from the maternal object, for he has remained attached to his mother as if he were one of her organs. On other occasions, the child plays the role of a fetish object, masking the Other's lack,[25] living evidence of a castration that has been denied. The treatment of a child cannot be undertaken without touching on the point where he is pinned down in the field of his mother's or father's desire.[26] The child has no choice in such circumstances, except to become the other's organ and deny as subject the necessity of being severed.

We have seen that the psychotic's fate is determined by the way in which he has been excluded by one or the other parent from the possibility of entering a triangular situation. It is that which dooms him to being incapable of ever assuming any identity. Trapped from birth in a flood of words that petrify him and reduce him to the condition of a partial object, the first prerequisite for his eventual participation in treatment as subject is a change in the system of language in which he is trapped. Only then does it become possible for him to be remodeled by language.[27]

[25] André Green, "L'objet (a) de J. Lacan," *Cahiers pour l'analyse*, No. 3 (May, 1966).

[26] A.-L. Stern, "Qu'est-ce qui fait consulter pour un enfant?" in *Relations affectives enfants-éducateurs*, Association Nationale des Centres Psycho-pedágogiques, day seminars, May 19–21, 1966.

[27] In the course of his development, the child is always in some way interwoven into his mother's demands. Insofar as he is, as a partial object, the stake of such demands, all words will bear on the partial object with which he identifies, and will arouse the anxiety that manifests his fantasy. If he accedes to the image of a unified body, it is as subject that he is the stake of the mother's demands. What

I have been guided in this study by the importance I attach to listening to *the only utterance*—that of the child and his family. I do not decipher a text in accordance with linguistic methods.[28] It is as an analyst (with my own set of problems) that I listen to what is being said in the unfolding of a personal history, which is changing or remaining petrified. The child is trapped in his parents' words that alienate him as subject. The alienating effect of a parent's words is one of the results of a symbolization that has gone wrong at the adult level. It is only when a word can free itself from impersonal discourse on the adult level that a different word from adult to child can emerge. The circumstances of the child's treatment are transformed from that moment. The type of communication I have described as "petrified" or "closed-circuit" appears in cases where the parent identifies with the analyst even as he cancels him out; the field in which his words operate does not open up any quest for truth. It takes several interviews to establish a prognosis, i.e., to weigh the chances of helping the parent bring about a confrontation between his Imaginary other and the third party (the locus where truth is articulated). If such a confrontation can occur only at the risk of the parent's death or an aggravation of his disorder, then there is little hope of curing the child. The alternative that decides the cure (either death or life for one or the other) is still more dangerous when it is unrecognized by the pathogenic parent; it is the chance he appears to have of assuming a truth "even at the risk of its killing him" (and in this case, it is an Imaginary death) that gives access to the words of drama. We then see the role played by the child as guarantee of the "unknowing" of the adult. He *is,* as the "sick" child, the prop of his own denial. In embarking on treat-

---

is implied in the castration threat, no longer brings the body into play—we are now entering verbal dialectics. We have seen how entering verbal dialectics appears to be barred to the psychotic at the beginning of treatment, and how, when he employs language, it is always to testify to his exclusion as subject.

28 I don't decipher archives; as an analyst, I listen to a drama. The remarks I carry away bear the imprint of my listening, that is, of how far I have been able to withstand being challenged through the tearing apart of the other's words.

ing the child, we touch on the parents' position in relation to words. The striking thing about closed-circuit communication is the *profession of faith* that accompanies it. The analyst is confronted with a belief that assumes the force of a *tabu*. If he touches it, he provokes breaking off the treatment, at best, and a paranoiac interpretation, even suicide, at worst.

The earliest results of Freud's findings regarding the approach to the problem of psychoses were revealed in the works of, first, Abraham, then Bleuler. Abraham had worked at Burghölzi and had been Bleuler's chief assistant. It would not be valid to say that Bleuler applied psychoanalysis to the problem of schizophrenia, yet he disagreed sharply with the views of psychiatrists of his day. Although he effected reforms in those views, he did not go as far as the psychoanalytic revolution would have allowed him to go. His attitude was *understanding* in the humanitarian rather than the scientific sense. The change of nomenclature to "schizophrenia" from "dementia praecox" is sufficient indication that he insisted on preserving Kraepelin's very rigid diagnostics and prognostics. Bleuler was less pessimistic and more liberal in the psychiatric approach to schizophrenia. In regard to the chances of cure he was an optimist, but he retained a pessimistic attitude towards the problem of therapeutic techniques. He even made the following astonishing remark: "The therapy of schizophrenia is most rewarding for the physician who does not attribute the results of a natural remission in psychosis to his own intervention." [29]

He had in any case an inkling of the importance of the part played by the word in schizophrenic families, but he did not push his investigations further. In the course of the last forty years, much has been written about the family of the schizophrenic, but in a sense in which the family is conceived as a group, or even as a biological organism. Furthermore, it is generally viewed in a pedagogical perspective.

---

[29] E. Bleuler, *Dementia Praecox or the Group of Schizophrenias* (New York, International Universities Press, 1950; London, Allen & Unwin, 1951), p. 471.

My research is linked to the actual direction of my cases and to the questions I ask myself about how to use words in psychoanalysis. Although I think I have highlighted the alienating effects on the child of the adult's words and demonstrated how treatment progresses by means of a change in language, I think I have not examined in sufficient detail the impasse created by the "closed circuit."

It is obvious that in having designated it by that term, I do not hold out any great hopes any longer for parents who seek out an analyst in order to exclude him from the communication going on in his presence. (This, of course, presupposes that I had greater hopes in the past.) My reaction is a subjective one, and it echoes failures that I found hard to bear. We probably ought to make an effort to rise above a certain form of self-justification, and it is likely that we would profit from a closer study of the nature of failures we have had with this type of parent. The analyst resents the exclusion he is subjected to, and reacts with his own personal problems. The technical difficulties we have encountered in certain cases should be studied in the context of our own contributions to the very blockages that we have observed.

PART 2

CHAPTER IV

PAUL, OR THE DOCTOR'S WORDS

Paul was on the verge of being hospitalized again at the age of two and a half. Suffering from anorexia and insomnia, he ruled the adults in the household with his symptoms. Did somebody venture to scold him? He fainted away. Was he given a tranquilizer? He developed sobbing spasms. His response to an attempt to feed him forcibly was an allergic attack. The mother admitted to being defeated. She was on the brink of nervous exhaustion. "The child has really got me down," she was to tell me.

The youngest of six children, Paul was born the day the oldest son was getting married. It had been an unwanted pregnancy. His mother obviously felt guilty at being pregnant once again at her age. From his birth, the baby had been cared for by an older sister and by more or less experienced outsiders. Nevertheless, by means of his symptoms, the baby made quite sure of keeping his mother at his side. In addition to his insomnia, he was prone to vomiting and suffered from a variety of nervous afflictions. The mother felt fenced in because she could not gratify her wish to be almost anywhere but where the child's needs kept her rooted. She responded to the demand for love by the gift of her care. In reality, Paul became the object of intensive nursing. Through it, he got to the stage of desiring *nothing* (which was the *total* gift of his mother), and that was where the source of his anorexia was situated.

Life in the home was organized (or disorganized) around Paul's claims; he had his mother at his mercy by his whims. She wore herself out, trying to satisfy the most contradictory desires. Paul would not stand for her being away, yet when she was there he refused everything from her hands. The father, kept out of the picture, avoided any sort of intervention.

When he was eighteen months old, his "convulsions" led to a psychiatric consultation. "The child will break you," said the doctor, "if you don't break him." At every attack, he was, in the mother's words, "stuffed with bromide." The child reacted by having an erection and masturbation. The doctor was consulted once again and explained to the mother (in front of the child) what caused the erection and the pain involved. "It's a frightful pain," he added. This comment touched off the mother's anxiety, and Paul remembered it. He woke up with an erection every night, called for his mother and said, "It hurts." Having imparted these words, he went back to sleep. It began to affect the mother's equilibrium, and the child was sent away for three months to a children's home. While he was there, he had no trouble sleeping, but stopped talking. Reunited with his family at the age of two and a half, he started to talk again, but stopped sleeping and refused food. In his fits of contrariness Paul felt injured—he would not allow his mother to pay attention to another child. Anxiety about being sent back to the children's home was expressed in increasingly frequent attacks of croup. His condition took a decided turn for the worse. "The child does not want to live. He must be put in the hospital at once," the doctor advised. The father opposed it, and it was he who was responsible for arranging a psychoanalytic consultation.

Occupied by his business affairs, the father did not attend the first two interviews; I had the mother alone. The mother's words centered around the theme of Paul's father. The child was very attached to him, yet scarcely saw him because the mother had a rigid routine that excluded Paul from their family life: "Since he is small, he must have a life apart. I'm always afraid of his getting the upper hand." The mother's anxiety crystallized around the imaginary danger of losing her authority (her power). Paul responded by demanding something which always left him unsatisfied. Every response in reality led to a further demand which could not be entirely satisfied. Paul enmeshed his mother in a web of contradictions. He concentrated his attacks around a refusal which was always the reverse side of an appeal. His father's failure to intervene, the fact that the child was not integrated into the pattern of home life, all worsened the effects of a dual situation. The rules the mother imposed were challenged as arbitrary; a battle for "prestige" was thus joined between mother and son; neither side wished to "yield," but then what would they have yielded? As far, and to the extent, that the mother came to realize the disorder in which she was participating, she perceived not only the lack of a triangular situation but also the importance of a parasitic factor in the link between herself and her son. *Paul could not lose his mother because his mother* (as a defense against the desire to abandon him) *could not lose Paul.* Therefore, no dividing line could be introduced. Everything went on as if Paul had never been weaned. Neither one nor the other could seize hold of a desire of his own, each lived by "pumping" the other. There was obviously no axis. My intervention dealt with the prohibition against parasitism; it introduced the emergence of the anthropophagic tabu and, at the same time, the idea of reference to a third. The form of my intervention was disputable, since it consisted in advice, although what I proposed was couched in the mother's words. She actually knew what was to be done but failed to recognize it. My words were aimed at a form of truth of which the mother already had a presentiment, as it were; I merely speeded up the outcome of events. I offered the following advice:

1. Complete freedom for the child insofar as it did not infringe on the others. (Freedom not to sleep, not to eat, not to wash, provided that no pattern of life "apart" was established to meet the child's whims.)

2. If Paul called out at night, I asked that it should be the father who got up and told him, "Do what you like, but leave me in peace with my wife. We must get some sleep."

The instructions were in the nature of an analytic interpretation, referring the mother to defenses linked to her Oedipal feelings of guilt. Paul's disorders vanished two days after his mother's interview with me.

"Who is your wife?" Paul asked his father in astonishment.

"Your mother."

"No, she isn't! She's my wife," the child replied.

An attack of croup subsequently caused a recurrence of the former disorders, and I agreed to see Paul.

He was small, thin, lively, and his big dark eyes seemed too large for his face. He was obviously very precocious. I saw him in his mother's presence and gave him a sort of briefing in adult language on his somatic ailments. I stressed the dual situation that existed between him and his mother, and pointed out how "inconvenient" the absence of language was for a baby. The child got off his mother's lap, looked at me in fascination, and launched into a long monologue of which I understood not a word.

"I should like to discuss all this with Daddy," I said to him.

"No," the child replied, "Paul is the big boss."

"No," I answered, "Daddy is the big boss. Mummy and Paul take orders from Daddy."

"No, no," the child contradicted me firmly, "Mummy is nice. Paul is Mummy's boss."

At the following session, ten days later, Paul proudly presented me with a letter from his father, in which he expressed his gratitude and recorded staggering progress on the plane of language. The child was now attending the local nursery school. Paul repeated to me in front of his mother, "Paul is the big boss. Daddy mustn't give orders." It was a game—at least, I considered it as such. The mother remarked that the child had been abandoned at birth: "I got rid of him through my daughter and the servants." Paul joined in: "It isn't nice not to sleep." I replied, "It isn't bad not to sleep, but it's inconvenient." The child again addressed me with an animated speech which I didn't understand much of, but which I recorded on tape. We agreed that it was unnecessary for me to see the family again, unless the father decided otherwise. Paul was not yet three; he was accepted as a full-day pupil in the local kindergarten.

Paul had used illness as a signal to awaken his mother's desire beyond her attentions in reality. He demanded that his mother gratify all his wishes, but at the same time he felt himself dispossessed as subject. He situated himself in their relationship sometimes in the place of Mummy's "big boss," sometimes in the place of sick little Paul. A certain relationship was structured *through pain* in a narcissistic mode. What Paul was offering his mother was not a penis in erection but *something that hurt,* and this began the day a "Doctor" explained the mysteries of an erection and its frightful pain to his mother. Paul retained from the explanation the possibility it offered, namely, the conversion of an organic manifestation into an illness. He set a value, not on the penis itself, but on how he could use it to appeal to his mother, the response to which was ready in the locus of her own lack. The child's regressive behavior occurred as a defense against castration anxiety. By bringing the father into the analytic interplay I helped the child to undertake the structuring of his Oedipal problem. He responded at first on the plane of his former defenses: "Mummy is *my* wife. Paul is Mummy's big boss," meaning, "I am, and I intend to remain Paul the tyrant, master of my mother's desire." By saying to the child, "Not sleeping hasn't got anything to do with not being nice; you sleep for yourself, not to give Mummy pleasure," I cut across the erotic mother-child link. When it was the father who answered the child's calls at night, Paul found himself on a circuit other than the dual relationship. Access to language became possible from the time the father intervened. The case illustrated the desirability of very early psychoanalytic consultation in emergency cases involving very young children. Psychosomatic symptoms reveal that transition from anxiety to symbolic expression is proving impossible.

So long as Paul was caught in his mother's words which left no room for reference to the father, he found it impossible to situate himself with regard to the object of his desire. What Paul demanded was the something else as such, namely, the forbidden. He was unable to embark on the dialectics of castration unless the mother was the one to bear its imprint. The doctor's words, "The child will break you, if you don't break him," in some way impelled the mother to freeze her relationship with the child in a narcissistic mode. "If you wish to keep the phallus," the doctor seemed to be saying, "on no account yield it to your son." Paul could not attain a phallic image on his own unless the mother was in a certain way dispossessed of it. Two homologous beings were locked in conflict in this child-mother confrontation, like the big giraffe and the little giraffe that Little Hans talked about. . . . The intervention by a father who owned Paul's mother enabled the boy to situate himself completely differently in the dialectics of desire. Access to language was opened to him by means of the mother's castration.

I received a progress report six years later which confirmed that Paul developed into an exceptionally gifted child; the psychosomatic weakness seemed to have disappeared.

Cases like Paul's are encountered every day in pediatric consultations.[1] A doctor's words always have a decisive influence.[2] They represent a confrontation between the doctor's desire and the parental anxiety. In this case, the doctor felt himself threatened in his being by the child's murderous-suicidal behavior. He defended himself by sanctioning the use of force which subsequently resulted in blocking any movement of the metaphor, thereby opening the door to the appearance of the symptom.

[1] Research carried out under the direction of Jenny Aubry (by R. Bargues, A.-L. Stern, G. Raimbault, et al.) bears witness to this.

[2] The doctor's words are easily distorted by the family; what we see then are the effects produced by the distortion.

CHAPTER V

CAROLE, OR THE MOTHER'S SILENCE

A very young couple was standing silently in front of me. They had come in behalf of their six-year-old daughter, Carole. The wife was holding her husband's hand. She was clearly under a strain, on the verge of tears. The man had adolescent features; he was unattentive and obviously distracted. The medical file sent to me by the hospital contained a diagnosis of schizophrenia (psychogenic muteness), and a recommendation that psychoanalysis was indicated. The mother was in a hurry for "something to be done." The father was resigned—they had had so many consultations with doctors "over the last four years. . . ."

"Not just over the last four years," the mother corrected him.

"What do you mean?"

"We were so young, barely out of high school. There I was, pregnant, with my studies to be carried on, and a future I mustn't jeopardize. I had to go on as if I hadn't been pregnant. Not even think about it, just become an automaton in order to keep my mind untrammeled. The birth came sooner than expected, and afterwards things weren't the same. Babies take up room, and she started being ill right away."

"Please explain."

"Carole was premature and she was born with jaundice. Then it cleared up and I managed to breast-feed her. I tried to arrange things so that I could study, but it wasn't easy. Four months later I was expecting again. I could have done without that. It got me down in the dumps. I was tired out and lonely. My milk stopped. I used to drag the baby around with me so that I could go on working. She got fussy and refused certain types of bottles. When she was six months old, I was told she had anemia. We had to work. We didn't get much in the way of help from anyone. I handed the baby over to my mother. I gave her, I took her back, then I finally handed her over again and I left her there until she was two years old. She got on well."

I learned that the child was not yet walking when her little sister was born. The two children were left with their grandparents. The young couple were facing difficult examinations as well as complicated professional lives. They both felt guilty about loving each other, and they did not know how to avoid pregnancies. The wife was hardly over the birth of her second child when she was pregnant again. She felt trapped in a vicious circle. She had to finish her studies at all costs. She had also to earn her living, and the children were too heavy a burden on her nerves. The husband hardly realized the strain such a life had been imposing on his wife. He was completely devoted to physics, and life seemed to hold no problems for him. Husband and wife did not talk to each other much, but they had a good understanding. The mother gradually relaxed during the interview. She needed to make the past relive itself for me. I learned that Carole spoke fluently at eighteen months. She was two when her mother took her back; she was happy to remove Carole from the grandparents' care. As soon as she was back home, the child became taciturn and sullen. She refused to eat anything. "She was simply letting herself die of hunger," the mother said. The surrounding world became more and more alien to her. She carried a headless, legless, teddy-bear with her everywhere. It had no more existence for her than her sister had. Carole walked all over it, squashed it, mistreated it. For a while, she was calling for her grandmother; then, she no longer asked for anything. "It happened without my noticing it. One day, she just didn't speak any more." When she stopped talking, Carole became phobic. She gradually regained her appetite, but she vomited at the slightest provocation.

The birth of the third baby did not improve things. Carole developed one little ailment after another, though none of them serious. When she was sent to nursery school, she ran off, and the school could not keep her on. "Her contact with human beings is severed," the mother remarked. "Carole plays with animals and stands daydreaming in front of flowers. Nobody knows what she thinks or what she wants. She takes no notice of us. A few words escape her, however, from time to time."

The father did not say much during the interview. He was in complete agreement with his wife. He was a little surprised, however, to see how emotional and intense she was about what she was going to *ask* me: "Tell me, is it true that you can give her back her speech? It hasn't gone for ever? And what if it doesn't work? Oh, yes, of course, you can't make any promises. Perhaps you don't know. Nobody knows what the matter is with her. I have been going from pillar to post. They say, 'Here are some tranquilizers you are to give her in the meantime.' "

"In what meantime?"

"Until she speaks—oh, I don't know. What I have just told you perhaps isn't what they told me. Perhaps I am misleading you. I mess everything up. I am tired out. I can't go on. I would like you to take charge of my child." [1]

At the end of the interview, the wife was unwilling to leave, she was crying. Gently, the husband led her away. It was clear that the mother, frozen and motionless at the beginning of the interview, now no longer knew where matters stood, nor where she was go-

---

[1] The mother believed that she had to "give up" the child, as she felt guilty about having "taken her back" from her own parents.

ing. "Psychoanalysis is required," the doctor had said to her; she had come to indict herself and "give up" her child to me. "Take charge of her," she begged. At the outset, she situated herself in a childish posture of guilt in relation to me, and she was astonished that I "gave her back" Carole, in order to take the child on as her own educator.

"I am a psychoanalyst," I told her. "It is only in that status that I can hear your past history, and your daughter's, and we shall see whether a meaning emerges." She came for advice to learn that she had to do the opposite—rethink her own life. "I don't love Carole," she said, "I have stood too much from her. No, that's wrong," she corrected herself, "Carole is my favorite. Can one prefer one child over another? I was the unloved one. I never did anything to make myself loved."

The young woman revealed in subsequent interviews her uncertainty, her anxiety, and her sense of a void which nothing had ever been able to fill. She wanted to be truthful, but the moment she spoke, her words betrayed what she had intended to say. She could express herself only through lies. Was the past as she had described it, or was it as she had presented it for her justification? Little by little, she let herself go, and ceased to be the frozen figure she had been at the first interview. Her husband came with her a few times, then she came by herself. It was at that stage that I decided to see Carole.

I saw the child sometimes in her mother's presence, sometimes alone. The mother kept herself in the background, though her eyes never left the child. Carole took no notice of me; she wandered around the room and stopped at the window to look at what was going on outside.

"Unless you ask her to do something, she won't do anything," the mother said.

I felt that the young woman was on edge. The child was playing with her braids. She had long blond hair. The short red pinafore she was wearing revealed thin legs imprisoned in ski pants. She was a graceful little girl, hopping from one foot to the other, ignoring our presence. I spoke to her, explaining who I was and why she was there. I talked to her at length about her past history, about that of her parents, and about the misunderstanding which had arisen without anyone's knowing why. The child sat down, picked up a red pencil, and traced some violent marks that tore the paper. She did two drawings for me. In one, a little girl had eyes but no mouth; in the other, a big circle rejected a small one. She tried to make me understand by gestures, then she would suddenly get up and go away. If I appeared to be asking something, she would go away also, but she refused to leave at the end of sessions when I had not *given* her anything. In effect, Carole was waiting to receive the true word, but she pretended to refuse it—or rather, she used her body as a prize, alternately offering and withdrawing it. From time to time, some words escaped her: "There's white rice outside." (She was referring to snowflakes.)

"No," cut in the mother, "those aren't the right words to use. What should you say?"

The child stared at me rebelliously with her big dark eyes, glanced at her mother, got up, and let go the words, "Ask the lady." Contact was broken again. Carole became absorbed in what was happening outside. I observed to the mother that when Carole did use words, the mother tried to substitute her own, instead. During the first eighteen sessions, Carole occasionally emerged from her muteness, adopting three types of communication. In one, she was spoken through by her mother. In another, she put a question from the locus of an imaginary adult in order to answer it from her own locus. In the third, she let drop a word or a phrase.

Carole had no wishes; a succession of fetish objects protected her from fear. When her mother was absent from a session, the child mimed her presence: "Show Madame M. Do this, do that."

"What is your very own wish?" I asked her.

Carole hid her face and replied: "Mummy."

This was a moment of revelation. Carole rarely used words, and never in order to make herself understood.

One day, Irene (the sister who was a year younger) came with her. Carole had insisted that she come. Irene drew, talked, walked about. Carole eclipsed herself completely; she had yielded her place. I pointed this out to her. Irene looked at me uneasily, but Carole did not bat an eye. She was conducting the game. The docile Irene continued to fill in the silence. What she said was of little importance; someone had to say something, and it was she who did.

Some time later, I saw Carole with her mother. The child was silent, obviously waiting for her mother to speak, but the silence remained unbroken by anyone. Carole got up, climbed on her mother's lap, and sucked on her thumb absent-mindedly.

"When Carole gets scolded," said her mother, "she does what I did as a child. She bites her wrist. I am sure that wrist is really me."

"Scolding isn't the same thing as eating," I replied (for Carole's benefit). "When a Mummy gets cross, there is a father inside her saying, 'Bring our daughter up well, take care of her.'"

Carole got up and pressed her face against the window. The mother wept. "Sometimes I get cross for nothing," she said in self-accusation.

The child left the window, a vacant expression on her face, as if she were sleep-walking, and threw herself on her mother, hugging her passionately. "You are my good Mummy."

The child was able to voice these words because I had appealed to the presence of the father in the mother. Carole did not feel afraid of being eaten (or of eating the Other) in a triangular situation. I had invoked in my intervention the figure of a father who lays down the law for both mother and child. At the end of this session, Carole left me her doll Marie, a trunk without head or limbs. She no longer wanted it. This fetish doll had been accompanying her for years wherever she went. She gave it up as soon as she discovered the disorder inside her own mother.

The next sessions were wordless. The child was drawing circles. "Those are Mummy's tummies," I said. "Once upon a time there was a father and a mother. They, too, were little once, and before them their parents also had parents."

I spoke in order to fill a period of silence. My impersonal discourse was like an incantation; there was no intention of creating a dialogue.

Carole kept looking for something shiny. She wanted to see her reflection in it. She was triumphant when she managed to find herself again in the mirror. She hid her face, turned away, gave a little jump, and jubilantly exclaimed: "It's Carole. She has found herself."

When Carole "found herself," she meant her tongue, her nose, or her braids. It was by them that she oriented herself—an expression of equivalence, also apparent in her drawings. She always gave people three legs or one. This had its beginning in the child's understanding during treatment that her mother was subject to the authority of a third party; she was then able to engage in this identification game, making use of parts of her body as recognition points.

"She was first deaf, then naughty. She seems happy now," the mother observed.

Carole was silently drawing stomachs, then attacking them. I said, "Carole wants all the good things that she thinks can come out of Mummy's tummy."

I subsequently verbalized the problem of Irene's birth and of the separations within the Oedipal framework. Carole listened to me without speaking, scribbling furiously. Throwing down her pencils, she turned to a puppet and murmured, "Indian hat."

The child then tried to "invest" the Indian hat in the mirror, as she had done with her tongue, her nose, and her braids. I emphasize again the possible meaning of this series of equivalences which reflected in her drawings of girls' bodies with one limb.

"Is the Indian cross?" asked Carole, and went on for herself rather than for me, "Prip, prip, he has come from a long way off, he has come and he says ba, be, bi, bo, bu."

Carole kept on the level of phonemes; as with the mirror, she tried to orient herself by a phallic signifier. More and more, the child was developing a private language; very chatty when she thought herself to be alone, silent when an adult approached.

When she tried to express herself, her throat tightened and precluded all possibility of speech. I said, "It's inconvenient not knowing whether Carole's words or Mummy's ought to come out."

The child took my hand and led me to a corner of the room where a piece of paper was lying which she had covered with crosses. "What's that?" she asked.

"They are what remain when people have disappeared. You can't blot out the traces," I said.

The child, panic-stricken, ran off to the bathroom. At the following session, with her mother there, Carole drew crosses. "They are graves," she said.

There were sobs from the mother, and then she talked about the death of her paternal grandmother. "It was to her I used to talk, not to my mother. . . . We went to Thionville for the anniversary of her death. The children did not know. Nevertheless, Irene commented, 'There have been baptisms and marriages, the only thing missing is a funeral.' "

When I was alone with Carole, I talked to her about what this grandmother had represented for her mother. "She was the wife of a man who liked your mother a lot." In response, the child, apparently indifferent, played with phonemes.

At home, she "came to life," provided no one took any notice of her. The mother told me, in tears, "Now I know what it means to be a mother; it means giving and not getting anything back in exchange. It means not expecting the child to make your own desires come true." Then she told me about her youngest child's anorexia. . . .

Carole made greater and greater efforts to speak. She tried to find terms to indicate what she observed: "That's a gnat, that's a light."

The Indian hat recurred in all the stories and stood for girls as well as boys and various phallic objects.

Carole started to ask her mother questions: "What are Mr. and Mrs. Hen doing?" No answer was expected, however. Words and questions were props for Carole. She was discovering herself through them.

In the transference relationship, Carole was clearly trying to make me be her motility, her words, her ears, and her nose. She accepted reluctantly the idea that she had to define herself as not alienated in me; between our bodies a complete game had come to signify her desire that I express with my nose what she smelled, that I draw with my hand the picture she had in her head. She attributed to me the power of reading her thoughts; a turning point was reached when she began to see that I could not guess her secrets. Carole was trying to establish a relationship with beings through separation. "There was once a grandpapa," she was to say to me a few weeks after the grandfather's departure.

It was a moment of intense emotion; through the "there was once" the child was in quest of all the lost objects of her babyhood —not only of the figure of her grandmother, but also of memories, such as the part played by the sense of smell in her relationship with her father. ("That smells of doodoo," was her way of saying "good morning" to him. The expression came back to her, as did another: "You have a parcel" meaning "I have done a doodoo, did you really smell it?") Carole was very eager to rediscover everything that reminded her of her babyhood. She appeared to mourn what was no more.

It was precisely at this juncture that the mother recollected, not in Carole's presence, her own failed dialogue with her father. She recalled a memory from the time she was five years old. "I didn't know him at all. He never spoke. One day I went into his study; I stopped short, panic-stricken. I got out two words: 'Daddy . . . shit . . .' and ran out."

The recollection of Carole's words as she offered her father the smell of her stools was particularly touching for the mother. In recalling this she said, "And I was always reproaching her, you mustn't say this, you mustn't do that, it isn't pretty, it isn't nice."

"Drawing her father's attention to the smell of her stools is a way of revealing herself as his daughter," I said. "You, too, offered yourself to your father as his daughter, but you panicked and ran away."

"Carole used to mean too much to me. I didn't want to know anything, I didn't want to understand anything. I had only one idea fixed in my head: to be stronger than my mother."

I then established with the child the parallel between the memories she had related to me and the mother's revelations, that is, the position of each in relation to the desire of the Other (the father).

"Where is O?" was the enigmatic question Carole asked at the next session. I recounted in an impersonal tone the story of Irene's birth. I prefaced it with the phrase "Once upon a time." The child got up. "Cuckoo, I am off," she said. Then, teasingly, she reappeared. "Cuckoo, when are you coming back?"

The affirmative statement in which the child assumed herself in the *I* (because she was disappearing) was followed by a question which the Other was meant to be asking her. "When are you coming back?" took the place of "I have come back." With the *I* she disappeared, with the *You* she came back, but it was the *I* that had disappeared.

We reached the fortieth session. At home and at school Carole used the word to express a desire, although she first tried to make herself understood by gestures. She consented to speak only if she failed to do so.

"My youngest is no longer suffering from loss of appetite," the mother told me. "You have transformed me. The two children were hostile to me because I was a tyrant. Since I no longer expect a reply from Carole, she is happy."

She wept and talked again about the absence of any dialogue with her mother. "There was nothing between us except a heavy silence."

Carole was making progress, but she was now offering herself in the form of various physical ailments (stomach aches, backaches, pains in her foot). She nursed herself with bandages and rubbing alcohol, and required hot water bottles and various attentions. She was looking for a symptom through which she could signify herself. This was taking place during a time when at other moments she complained that "she lacked something." What? She didn't ex-actly know. Scowling and disgruntled, she wandered around in search of what could not be given her. She cried easily, was hard to please and capricious. Increasingly, her mother came to represent for her the one to whom she talked, and her father the one from whom she received caresses. The mother's parents appeared in a new light for her. Through her mother, Carole discovered in the person of her grandfather the image of a respected authority on whom the mother concentrated her feelings of bitterness. There was a grudge against him, and for that reason he acquired a certain prestige in the child's eyes. She then situated herself in the conflict that divided her mother from her grandparents and had made her the stake in a jealous love, the representation of what the mother had not received from her own father. In removing Carole from the grandparents' affection, the mother had failed to observe one of the rules of the game, that is, a third party must preside over all such exchange operations. This third party, in the person of the husband, had been kept out of the picture by the mother, after she had limited his role in the person of her father. The child, in con-fusion, no longer knew on whose side she could take her stand. Only the preservation of a triangular relationship could have pro-tected her from the danger of being so dominated by the mother as to be forced to give up having words of her own. During the treat-ment Carole witnessed her mother's struggle to become aware of her own rejection of the paternal image. This made it possible for the child to remodel the signified; an anxiety crisis began which was to indicate new possibilities of reorganization, first of all on the level of language.

The child took pleasure in the grammatical discoveries she was able to make, and never stopped talking about problems of tense in the use of verbs. "She is going to leave it, she has left it; they are quite different," she said to me thoughtfully.

Whenever Carole felt herself to be in danger, or when she was merely depressed, she hastened to find herself again in the mirror.

"With this body I have rediscovered I can talk to you again," she seemed to be telling me. Nevertheless, Carole still appeared to experience difficulty in identifying with a reflection of herself; consequently, she had a considerable problem about undertaking the dialectics of identifying with the Other. Jealousy of Irene was thus denied, and the *I* and *You* were occasionally mixed up. While Carole could use words at this stage, she was not yet cured. The current theme in treatment was the impression of danger which all her encounters with the Other seemed to arouse.

Carole's treatment had been conducted on two levels—the mother's (interviews with the mother alone), and the child's (interviews with the child, first in her mother's presence, then alone). Through the indirect means of her daughter's symptom, the mother came to spontaneously revaluate her own position.

At first she came with her husband. She needed his presence as a guarantee against fear. By expressing a phobic anxiety, the young woman was impelled to tell me about her own Oedipal problem, and her jealousy. On the fantasy plane, she apparently situated herself in relation to her own family as the child who had been excluded and little loved, which created a situation that was not conducive to any dialogue between herself and her parents. Carole's mother was unconsciously repeating a situation from her own childhood in that she had put her husband in the place of one from whom she did not expect to receive any words; she proposed to receive them from her daughter.

The more she overwhelmed Carole with demands and needs, the more the child slipped away from her. It was from the nothingness in which she had lost herself that she then seemed to be addressing an appeal for love to her mother. In return, she got solicitude weighed down with unreasonable demands. The mother's dissatisfaction could never be remedied. She herself perceived this one day in a flash of illumination. "It was me," she said, "who created the situation where my oldest child doesn't talk and my youngest doesn't eat."

She made this admission after introducing the figure of her paternal grandmother for whom, without knowing it, she still mourned. The grandmother represented the image of one to whom one could speak, in contradistinction to all others, particularly her father, whom she perceived as hostile. After this admission she brought up matters that had been in the domain of the unsaid: her death-wishes, her jealousy. The child, in her symptom, had to some extent made herself their representation.

This admission was a discovery for the mother; afterwards, she no longer felt the need to beg words from her oldest child, and Carole's muteness began to yield while the anorexia of the youngest disappeared.

Although Carole gradually recovered the use of words, she was, as we have seen, far from being cured. The work with her mother was carried on in an analytic dimension. The young woman discovered, among other things, that she was not able to be a mother because as a child she had evaded the issue of Oedipal rivalry while endeavoring to assert herself as the favorite. "I never spoke to my parents," she said, "and words don't come to me with my child. It is as if I had none to give."

The mother "masked" her confusion by making ever increasing demands on her children, particularly on the oldest. In her relationship with Carole, she prevented the birth of any *desire* by a game in which she tried to substitute her own words and demands for the child's. Her recognition of these problems made the parallel treatment of the child much easier.

The mother's presence made it possible for me at the beginning to grasp a total physical game in which the mother asserted herself as the owner of her child's hair, hands, and feet. Carole arrived at one session with her hair windswept, her shoelaces untied, and her overalls unbuttoned. In a twinkling, the impeccable grooming of a model child had been re-established. "I don't like to have hair in my mouth," said the mother, "and I would fall with my laces untied."

I attempted to introduce in words what I perceived at the level of this sharing of mother-child body. My interpretation, which emphasized the existence of two different bodies and wishes, caused confusion and embarassment in both mother and child. I was the third party who risked impeding relationships of a certain type.[2]

In Carole's case, we have seen that the child asserted her existence through the indirect means of *non-demand*. She shared her body, in turn, with Irene, her mother, or another adult. An automaton, she escaped us; she seemed to be looking back at us from the very locus of her flight, from where a word occasionally reached us.

At first, she let fall only impersonal chatter; then she maintained herself on the level of phonemes; finally, she attempted correct enunciation. She tried to use appropriate tenses, she was concerned with grammar. The contrary use of *I* and *You* seemed to be associated with difficulties in establishing identification with the Other's image. Carole's mirror-play seemed to indicate that she was looking for an unmutilated image of herself. When she found herself again in the mirror, it was in effect to signify herself in a phallic signifier (tongue, nose, or braids).

In the field of *communication,* her speech was at first a *private language,* a play with words meant for herself alone. Next, when Carole first attempted to address the Other, her throat tightened and made all dialogue impossible. By touching on the signifiers "father," "death," "phallus" in the child's treatment, a question was brought to light which had originally arisen in the mother; it was therefore as a function of what was going on in the mother that the child sought to orient herself and got trapped.

We have seen that Carole represented her mother's disorder in her symptom. As soon as the mother found herself able to put into words something of the order of the unsaid, the unconscious mother-child relationship altered, and the effects of this were felt in the words. Verbalizing the mother's Oedipal problem was the key to the treatment; from that juncture, the real child was able to express a desire. Carole acquired a value as soon as her mother

[2] I obstructed the establishment of a dual relationship.

could recognize in her own father what lay beyond that which was repressed by the child. Before, there was nothing beyond that; the little girl found herself alone, confronted with a devouring Other.

In the course of treatment, interpretations turned fundamentally on the phallic signifier, on death, and on the present-absent play. We then saw the appearance of signs through which the child was trying to ask herself what the Other required of her. The trouble was that all questioning about the Other's desire plunged her into panic; she sought to reinvest a partial image of herself—and at the same time, specific, clearly differentiated child-father and child-mother attitudes were becoming established. The child's relationship with her father was wordless. Yet, Carole tried to convey through him to her mother the love he showed her, subsequently finding a possibility of dialogue with her mother through negation.

In sum, Carole's muteness was structured on the model of anorexia. There was no chance of symbolization for the child so long as the mother was seeking a response in reality to her own basic dissatisfaction.

I did not try to bring out the fantasy elements in this treatment. My work was concerned with uncovering a certain failure of recognition in the mother which had brought about a complete loss of orientation and words in the child. Because certain questions about her father, sex, and death could not be posed to herself by the mother, the child found herself trapped in trying to articulate her demands by her relation to the mother's desire. This posture of the subject—panicked by any attempt at symbolization—was propped up by the mother, and that was why I listened so attentively to her words.

We were able to situate the start of the child's difficulties in the weaning period. It was noticed at the age of four months that the baby seemed to be withering away,[3] withdrawing her investment in her body, which subsequently caused the difficulty with her

---

[3] Weaning coincided with the mother's second pregnancy, probably perceived by the baby from that juncture.

mirror-image. In effect, Carole's eventual engagement in the dialectics of the relationship with the Other was to be undertaken with the image of a body "in bits and pieces." The unease that followed weaning took the form of a fundamental masochism in Carole. She wavered between moves of violence and a sort of desire to let herself die. She would habitually bite herself; the doll she dragged around with her was but a mutilated trunk. Carole had no mastery over her emotions, and any Imaginary mastery was foredoomed. The problem of jealousy was lived through an alternative where her non-existence was face to face with the existence of the other (the Imaginary other). When Carole *recognized* herself in her body, the other was to be suppressed or ignored.

All relations of the child to the Other during the first phase appeared as a wavering between a desire to co-operate with other people, and the wish to remain separate, unrecognized as subject. To use words, to feed herself, to live or to die were all activities belonging in one context, and it was from there that the child signified to us the difficulties in which she was floundering. The development of the treatment was marked by a twofold movement. We saw the child wavering between finding her image in the mirror, and the effort to sustain her question in face of an Other perceived as dangerous and devouring. A transference relationship was established with me *through* the mother, for whom I became the support of anxiety and the repository of so-called bad or dangerous thoughts. Once the mother got over a certain failure of recognition of which the child was the instrument, she was able to establish a correct relationship with the child. The mechanics of the cure threw light on the meaning of the role of mediator, which I played in the treatment, as grasped by mother and child.

We began with what had been a dual situation. The mother's admissions about her childhood then introduced the figure of a prohibitory father whose law the mother had rejected. At this juncture in the treatment, I was an embarrassing third presence. Later, the mother made the connection between what she had rejected in her Oedipal history, and what she had been unable to symbolize in her relations with her child. Echoing a question the mother could now ask, Carole introduced the notion that she lacked something. My position as the third presence between mother and child now shifted imperceptibly from being embarrassing to being permissive. I became the mediator in the sense that it was through what the child refused me that she could use the word with her mother, and it was through what the mother revealed to me that she enabled Carole to express herself.

Although the mother-child relationship was changed, it would be false to say that my role in the analysis had consisted in being an interpersonal link. By bringing to light what was unsaid in mother and child, I referred each to her own system of signifiers. Trapped as they were in a highly neurotic situation, the part played by each became clear during the treatment, casting light for the child on the meaning of a symptom that had become the only locus where she could signify herself as subject. The analyst's function was something other than to correct deficient parental figures, as the deficiency to be corrected was not at all on the level of the ego. In fact, there was no deficiency on the Imaginary plane; what Carole's mother had to reintegrate was a Symbolic repression. The return of what had been repressed in the pathogenic parent opened the Symbolic track for the child. The child had to recognize herself within a certain structure, and she conveyed right from the start that she would use the word only to define herself according to what her mother wished to assume or reject in her own past history. When the mother was able to reveal the forgotten words "Daddy . . . shit," which implied emphasizing the dimension of rejection in her own Oedipal history), the child felt herself entitled to remodel the signified, and to give a meaning to what had been blocked under the web of meaninglessness where her mother had been holding her prisoner.

The mother's unconscious wish was not to recognize her daughter in the line of descent from her father, that is, not to recognize her as subject of desire. She thereby condemned her daughter to re-enact her own refusal to pay her debt to her father, and perpetuated not only an unpaid debt but, worse, a self-refusal to exist.

Carole, by her muteness, her sister, by her anorexia, had been indicating unmistakably that there was an unanswered question in the mother's own past history: Was I born desired or not? It was in this mode of being that the mother gave birth to her own children —in uncertainty as to whether they were brought into the world to live *or* to die. The mother was enabled through my analytic listen-ing to establish a situation in which her children no longer had to enact her personal problem. This was sufficient to bring the younger child out of the anorexia in which she had taken refuge. As far as Carole was concerned, she was given time to resume on her own the questioning of her mother. She perceived through analysis where her mother's problem lay. She embarked on some-thing on the order of the Oedipal problem, having first become reconciled with the ancestor whose mantle had fallen upon her in her mother's eyes. It was to some extent in the name of that father in the past that Carole was able to become loving daughter to the father in the present. So long as the child embodied in the present the disowned father for the mother, she did not have the means to bring to life what was clamoring to speak in her. Analysis of the mother eventually opened the door for her children to a solution other than suicide.

CHAPTER VI

GUY, OR THE FATHER'S DEATH

At the hospital I was asked to examine the case of six-year-old Guy. The diagnosis of retardation seemed incontestable, but there were views to the effect that a schizophrenic factor contributed an integral part to the clinical picture. There was general agreement on the gravity of intellectual deficit. The school refused to keep Guy. The mother, always clad in black, trailed her child from one department to another, and kept on asking what they wanted from her. The welfare officer persuaded her, not without difficulty, to "do something." It was difficult to establish the history of the disease. The mother had nothing to say. "The boy is unstable, but no one noticed anything until he went to school."

The replies were dragged out of her one by one. Time was needed to gain this woman's confidence.

"I can't do anything for you," I said. "Come back when you and your husband have decided to do so yourselves. After all, he is your child, not the welfare officer's."

Madame X began to weep silently. "If it isn't to put him away, I'm quite willing. I'm always afraid they'll take him away from me."

The interview continued, still very much uphill. I felt I was dragging the words out one at a time. The child had been un-wanted, his motor development had been very slow. He was not allowed even to stir; his father could not stand it.

The father was a skilled workman who was on the nightshift at the time. He had to sleep during the day, which was not easy to arrange in a two-room apartment.

Guy's parents got on well. They had occasional quarrels about the child. The father was very exacting and the mother protected him. She said nothing about her own family. I learned that her husband's mother had been hospitalized several times with attacks of "melancholia." Guy's father was very attached to his own mother; on the other hand, he was very angry at his wife's parents and had ordered her to break with them. I was to learn no more at the first interview.

Enter Guy. He had big blue eyes and a shock of blond hair. He was big, well built, and solidly planted on his feet. He didn't stand still but went from one object to another in a sort of feverish haste. He held a monologue: "The dickie is broken, the witch makes poison, the bee will eat her."

The child drew something (scribblings in red pencil), seized the modeling clay, ran out, got lost in the corridors, then came back. He sat down and started up again without drawing a breath: "It's a cock. It wants to eat the wolf. That's the way with the wolf, kill him, bang, he's dead. They cut his head off. They make a fire. They burn him. They kick his mouth in. They eat him. They make a big fat spider. She is nasty. Father Christmas has gone off to eat some meat. They put his eyes out. They make sausages with the dog's tail."

Guy never once addressed me. There were crayons and modeling clay available; he had been told previously to use them. Like an automaton, he drew, talked, and modeled. Words went spinning around and there was a procession of severances. "They" did this, "they" did that—who? No one knew. Guy had apparently taken cover. Between him and myself there was some real object he gave me (a drawing, for one) and that, he thought, was what I was asking for. Any questioning caused him anxiety. His fantasy out-pouring was a form of protection. He had no use for dialogue.

I saw the mother again. She confirmed that the difficulties did not start until Guy entered school. "Before, Guy was no problem. As soon as he began to walk he was stopped from touching things. He was stopped from doing anything so that he didn't disturb his father."

In effect, since the age of three months the child's needs had brought death. (He was given barbiturates to stop him from cry-ing; the father could not endure a living child.) The fear-stricken mother tried to stifle any awakening to desire in the baby. Above all, the child must not disturb the father. There was no question about it, the phrase recurred like a *leitmotiv*. I was not to grasp its implications until later.

Psychoanalysis was suggested and the father's consent was re-quested in writing, as we couldn't manage to see him. I made the mistake of giving way to a *real* argument; there was a money prob-lem and the father found it impossible to come. I allowed myself to be convinced by the mother: "My husband needs his sleep. He can't leave his job. He'll come later, but not now."

The letter in which the father gave his consent was a downright appeal for help *for his son,* masking in effect the father's own con-fusion. He confirmed that circumstances made it impossible for him to keep an appointment.

I should have insisted on at least one meeting, but I did not. I should have probed more deeply into the meaning of the father's "tiredness," and into the "rest" that had to be safeguarded ever since Guy's birth. If the child started treatment, might it not bring into play a sort of alternative: If Guy is to get well, is the father to die of it? In the words I wrung out of the mother, I should have paid greater heed to the one false note—the place assigned in the family life to the father's tiredness. The mother spoke in a dis-jointed, monosyllabic way. It was the social welfare system, not the

157

needs of the family, which had initiated this consultation. The mother had the feeling that she could no longer evade a form of moral pressure. "Something really must be done for the child." The diagnosis of mental retardation, which had been made repeatedly, did not scare her. Had she not grown up with a younger brother who was backward and difficult?

The theme of the first three months of treatment. The child would tell a castration story associated with things he had seen or heard, or a story directly linked to the primal scene. His fundamental theme emerged in various permutations and combinations. The mother would be represented in the shape of a witch who oozed poison. The child's hatred was directed against her. The witch (who was mad) had a man who beat her regularly. The child chose to remain with the father (but the father's cock was smashed). Elements Melanie Klein has illuminated were clearly recognizable—aggression against the father is displaced onto the mother's stomach, it being the receptacle containing the father's penis, and the mother is *seen as* dangerous because she swallows the father's sexual organ and emits poison around her.

"A wolf had a feast on the boy's broken dickie. The wolf enjoyed it all right, but it killed the boy. A witch made poison. It's food to her, you have to be careful. There, that's the Gentleman's cock. She smashes it. Nasty witch, she gives poisoned apples while the animals fuck around."

In transference, the child put me in the witch's place and formed the wish that I die. He imputed to me the role of castrator and accused me of breaking apple stems. "A cigarette lighter is a man's thing," he added. "You have no right to have one."

The child identified with a series of partial objects, and he was unable to situate his desire anywhere but in death. Destructive drives appeared in the place of incestuous desire. It was on a note of death-wish (for me) that Guy departed for his vacation. The fantasy theme he had brought up was a primal scene involving death. "Mammy and Pappy died of making love; they joined themselves together and then they didn't stir any more. They were dead."

Eight days after Guy had left for a sanatorium (it was his first time away from home), *the father committed suicide.* The mother told the child about the father's death two months later. "Daddy's in the cemetery, we will take him some flowers." The child, his expression wooden, flinched, then pulled himself together and said calmly, "There's no such thing as death; it isn't true that Daddy's dead." *It was as someone who did not know* that his father was dead that Guy established himself in his relationship to the Other.

On his return from vacation he came to see me and went to the telephone, saying, "I'm going to 'phone my parents, because there must be three people, two isn't right."

Thus the child became a subject of desire from the baseline of death. But the phrase seemed to be out of context. He was again detached from reality. Indifferent to objects, he retired into a hostile silence.

At this point, the maternal grandmother came into the picture. She turned up one day with her daughter. It seemed impossible to separate the two; a hand on her daughter's shoulder, the old woman strode firmly forward. "Now that my son-in-law is dead, it is my duty to take his place. My daughter is at a loss. She is incapable of deciding things for herself. Guy must be put in an institution so that his mother doesn't worry about him. In our view, it would improve her state of health. We will not leave our daughter on her own. If Guy had not had such a difficult childhood, we would have taken him, but we don't want to have him. The father's death has been a blow to the family. We will not stand idly by while there is a risk of the mother's death, too."

The grandmother spoke loudly and clearly, she was apparently conscious of her role as head of the family. Guy's mother wept silently, completely crushed under her mother's authority. She had just lost her husband and they were asking her to give up her son. Guy must pay for his father's suicide, they seemed to be saying. I asked the grandmother to leave me alone with her daughter: "Your daughter does not need you. I have a letter from Guy's father, asking me to treat him. His wish is to be respected."

The grandmother departed, outraged. Her daughter, relieved of her presence, slowly recovered her spirits, and then told me about the struggle that has raged between the female line and the male line in both families, generation after generation. The women had money, but they always married beneath them. Guy's father, in contrast to his own father, was a hard worker; he provided for his family and supported his mother (a woman who was forever complaining). The maternal grandmother taunted him with his "low birth" and never forgave him for the hold he had over her daughter. Guy's mother associated him with a backward boy (like her own brother), but to the grandmother he was insane—"like his father's mother, and he'll die raving. If my daughter keeps him, she'll be next to commit suicide." Now that her son-in-law was dead, the grandmother reverted to her dream (the expression of the family myth) of having her daughter make a "good" marriage. The only obstacle was Guy.

The father's death. Guy was again threatened with being sent away. He became overbearing and rebellious at school and at home. "For me, it's as if everything were just the same as before," the mother said to me.

I confessed that I didn't understand. She decided to talk, and described the hell she had lived in. Her husband used to beat her every night, demanding that she tell him the names of her lovers. Towards the end, he became taciturn, refused food, and became obsessed by the idea that his wife was poisoning him. His son got on his nerves. He never got over the fact that he had "made a living being." Yet, he loved the boy, the mother said. "He had high hopes for psychotherapy. He used to say to me over and over again, 'I don't want Guy to get to be like me.'"

The drama of Guy's father consisted in his obligation to pay the debts incurred by his own father and in the necessity of providing for his mother. In his turn, he left it for Guy to face his debts along with those of the boy's grandfather. But, as we have seen, Guy had established himself as someone *who did not know* that his father was dead. (In his behavior, he appropriated the insignia of the father who disappeared; meanwhile, his mother regained some words of her own.)

Guy set himself up to judge: He demanded his father's return, and at the same time accused his mother of having poisoned him. I explained to him that it was not so. "I know that your Daddy was ill. The false sick Daddy is dead. The real Daddy lives in your heart. He is happy that the false one can rest in peace, at last. The real Daddy loved you and wanted you to grow up and become the next Mister X. You bear the name of all the men of the family."

"You filthy little thing," Guy replied, "I shall go on asking for my Daddy back."

"Filthy little thing" was the equivalent of "darling." A partial object has become a possible support for a subject to the child. He was trying to build himself up as subject in the guise of *loss,* but sought to deny the very existence of desire in the Other, namely, the existence of castration.

The theme of the primal scene reappeared in all the child's fantasies. "The house committed a mortal sin. It fell down. The lady sinned with the gentleman. They went to bed, and Punch leaped into the air."

Incestuous desire, perceived more and more clearly, accompanied the destructive drives directed against his mother. The child claimed objects that had belonged to his father, but if someone spoke of him, Guy ran away or used scatological language. During this entire phase of treatment, Guy presented himself as a partial object; he *was* the pee, the doodoo of someone *in the style of his father* (the partial object of his melancholy mother). Session after session, it went on like a phonograph record, "pee, doodoo, bathroom, Punch."

One day, I intervened. "You keep putting pee and doodoo between us as if you wanted to believe that Daddy-Mummy are just pee and doodoo talking. Doodoo is what is left over from what you eat. Are you just a leftover from Mummy and Daddy? What are you getting at? You are a living child."

Guy manifested a desire in school to write, but in our sessions it was the word of the sick father that was transmitted through him: "You're a slut. You're the whore of the neighborhood."

I tried to find out with him what he recalled about his father before the latter's illness. (In effect, it was a device to help the child symbolize what was valuable in the father.) Guy's response came a few days later: "I won't be called Guy, Robert, Martin."

These were the Christian names of the father and grandfather. He thus expressed the wish of not getting well in relation to a destructive father figure. "I'm poisoned. Daddy-Mummy did it to me."

It was the parents' desire that Guy not be born to desire. He wavered between various identifications. In transference, I became one who was the victim of men and he, too, was a victim. Then, a dilemma was reached: If he identified with the mother, he received death from the father; if he identified with the father, his sexual organ was infertile, because it had been his father's desire not to bring him into the world. How to be born from such a primal scene? This was the problem which was to weigh Guy down for nearly a year.

"I don't want to be a dead Daddy," he said to his mother.

At other times, he defended his disappeared father; it was his way of mourning him. "My Daddy is dead. He didn't want you any more, so he did silly things." And: "My Daddy is dead. He ate poison. Daddy had a depression. You are weaving me into your spider's web," he said to his mother.

Guy knew about his father's death while rejecting it. He brought to the sessions words of adults concerning the suicide. The words were transmitted through him, he did not assume them. At the end of the second year of treatment, the child made two admissions:

"I don't love my Daddy any more, because he isn't coming back."

"When people bother me, I act crazy."

At the same time that he accepted being marked by the Loss of the Father, Guy admitted that he *acted crazy,* he was playing at it. The game turned out badly, for the special school he was going to did not want to keep him any longer. He was hospitalized. The grandmother demanded nothing less than that he be committed. The entire family and the pressure of society suddenly formed an alliance against the child.

Fully aware of what was happening Guy then explained to the doctor that it was his teacher (at that time in a depressive episode) who had made him crazy, and he expressed the wish to get better. This wish was linked to the acceptance of his own death, and it marked a turning point in treatment. "If I get better, I could die."

The child vacillated between the idea of accepting that he was mortal—and, as such, subject—and the idea that the Other's desire was driving him back to being only a partial object. "When I'm shouted at, it's as if the voices of all the daddies in the world were demanding my arms, my legs, and all that."

The child was trapped in the words of adults who were trying to remove him from the reach of psychotherapy. He hung on: "I must get better, grow old, and die."

He reclaimed his family name, but he was no longer prepared to put up with the dual situation with his mother. She became depressed. All the scenes she had had with her husband came back to her; she told me how the child had taken her part, saying to his father, "You leave my mother alone."

The child was boarded out with a foster family long enough for the mother to recover. On his return, he took possession of the house, as if he were his mother's man, and announced that he was going to give her a child. This constituted the culminating point of the "illness." Guy had to renounce identification with his "sick" father, with his mother, and with his incestuous desire. We reached the end of the third year of treatment. Guy had become very fond of a family friend. The man died, and it was through the child's mourning for him that he consummated the mourning for his father, and declared himself cured.

Nevertheless, I continued to follow the case, for every time the child made progress, the mother fell into another depression, sending him back to his place as "sick." One day, she came to see me. "We must board Guy out; he's killing me."

The child went back to the foster family, which he esteemed, and the mother was given medical attention. One day, she asked to see me again. "I had an awful dream. I saw myself scalding my brother, but the brother was Guy."

It was after this admission—which she made after having expressed the fear that Guy would kill her—that the mother came to the acceptance of her child's assumption of his own word. The brother she was referring to was a younger brother whom she had killed through clumsiness; the fact that she associated him with Guy pinpointed the place she assigned to the latter in her own Oedipal problem: the place of the retarded brother, or that of the dead one. Becoming aware of all this was to be a turning point for the mother; she soon took a job she liked, started to have a life of her own, and agreed to keep the child with the foster family. Guy, relieved of his mother's presence, made spectacular progress. He found identification with the foster father, and told his mother: "I hope you are going to get married some day. You can't go on as you are."

Guy repeated his conviction that he was cured. He didn't want to stay in a "school for abnormal children" any longer, and wanted to be apprenticed to a friend who was a plumber.

His I.Q. was still low and bore out the original diagnosis of mental retardation. His educational attainments were rudimentary—he could read, write and count, and that was all. He was very good with his hands, and was highly regarded by adult artisans and workmen. In the world of work, he was considered reliable and handy. (In the country, the child used to help the baker and accompany the plumber on his rounds.) The men in his family were bakers, carpenters, or plumbers; it was very much in keeping with his father's insignia, as it were, that Guy proposed to integrate himself into life. He was able to do this as soon as he accepted that he was *mortal*. From then on, he was trying to orient himself in relation to a Law, having renounced his anthropophagic and incestuous desires through his mourning for structuring father figures. The part played by the foster family was important; for the first time, the child was living with non-alienating familial words. He has made sufficient progress in his analysis to gain from it.

In the course of the treatment, Guy successively utilized an *impersonal* discourse (the father's word or the mother's complaints), the *language of tales* (relating stories as if they did not concern him), and, at last, *his own word,* beginning with the wish to see me dead. To the extent that his word asserted itself, we came up against familial words that sent him back to non-being or to remaining insane.

During the treatment we have seen the following stages: (i) The child had no choice but to situate himself as partial object in his relation to the Other. At that point, he denied the existence of death and of castration. (ii) Various permutations of the initial theme of the primal scene had taken place throughout the sessions. Guy's closed-circuit responses were made through these, and they had to be challenged. This led to Guy's inquiries about his right to existence. (Guy was indeed born through his father's death, and to live at such a cost is a heavy load for a child to bear.) (iii) Guy finally acquired the right to live by facing the unpaid debts of his father and grandfather. He paid for the crime of existing by renouncing his mother and by choosing to be mortal (but without any desire of suicide). He ended by renouncing identification with the suicided father as well as with his mother. He acceded to desire as soon as he accepted the fact that the object of his desire (his mother) was barred by interdiction. After that, he found himself again as subject, marked by symbolic castration. (Previously, any idea of castration was foreclosed.)

If we follow the same line of development in the *transference,* it was as "filthy little thing" that I first became the possible prop for a subject. Then we went into a series of permutations on the identification plane. The child's fantasies referred back to the parents' murderous words. We have seen how Guy was shaped by them. An alienated word re-echoes alienating discourse. *Guy could not be born from the primal scene.* The situation was challenged through the play of transference, that is, in relation to the Other's desire. What the child's anxiety revealed was a threat from the Other, coupled with a danger of physical injury.

If the child's drawings made in the course of analysis showed progression, it is because he acquired insight into the very meaning of his desire through the play of the signifier. In his fantasy theme, the child indicates that there is a mask; it is beyond this that the pawns on the chessboard have to be moved into new positions, in accordance with a rule which is that of the order of language itself. We are involved in a dialectics where the relations of the subject with his own body are paramount. The child's relations with the image of a partial body, or of a unified body of himself, outline his type of relationship with the Other and offer an understanding of the permanent role to be played by the castration fantasy in his experience. If he does not have an image of a unified body of himself, he will always be faced with the Other's desire, in danger of being rejected, because he is totally identified with the object of demand. It seems probable that in the course of his development, the child is always woven into his mother's demands in some way.[1] Insofar as he is, as a partial object, the stake of such demands, the exigencies of society will bear down on the partial object with which he identifies, arousing the anxiety which is manifested in his fantasy. If he does accede to an image of a unified body, it is as subject that he is the stake of the mother's demands, and he will be able "to assume castration," i.e., to understand that the test to be undergone does not bear on the totality of the subejct. It seems as if at a certain juncture the implied contents of the castration threat no longer brought the body into play—we are now entering a verbal

[1] See footnote 27, Chapter III.

dialectics. We witness in the progression of a treatment a series of permutations which indicate, when re-articulated into the analytic speech, what had been introduced behind a mask. It is from the very locus of his fantasy that the subject comes to understand how he situates himself in relation to the Other's desire.

Guy questioned the image of his dead father at various junctures before situating his desire; as we have seen, he found desire only at the cost of recognizing himself to be mortal. From the time he learned about his father's suicide, the child clung to the insignia of all fathers by way of their shortcomings. Could I have prevented this suicide?

The matter is certainly worth examining. Since I had not met the father, I was not in a position to evaluate the meaning of his desire. The appeal for help *for his son* could very well have been an appeal for help for the child within himself who had not succeeded in coming to life. My mistake lay in not knowing how to read the message addressed to me. I became the involuntary accomplice in a death-wish. The medical report on Guy's father (who was hospitalized before his suicide) refers to the appearance two months previously (one month after Guy began treatment) of a syndrome of frenzied jealousy. He improved after a course of chemotherapy and left the hospital, only to commit suicide immediately.

The outcome might have been different if the child had remained "ill," or if I had suggested putting off treatment. Nothing entitles us to assume that this ending was ineluctable.

CHAPTER VII

MIREILLE'S QUESTION

My goal here is to examine closely a type of speech used by a child who in posing her question could but pose the question of another, in this case, that of her father.

The parents were referred to me by Dr. X. who had recommended psychoanalysis for their eight-year-old daughter, Mireille, the second of five children. The diagnosis was "schizophrenia against a background of mental retardation." A few months earlier, two other specialists had singled out "feeble-mindedness" and suggested glutamine treatment together with special training in orientation.

The medical file contained the following: (i) Details of the child's previous disorders. (Agoraphobia at the age of two and a half, following the birth of her sister Carole and a separation from the family; coprophilia and exhibitionism at the age of five, following a traffic accident; retardation diagnosed at age five, and schizophrenia at age eight. The mother stated that the child's development from birth to age two and a half had been normal.) (ii) A copy of the report from the hospital where Mireille was taken for a short while as a result of her accident. She had suffered slight head injuries. The child was unstable and easily upset, and she disturbed hospital routine; she was released with a diagnosis of mental retardation plus associated character disorders. (iii) A copy of the decision of the Medical Control Board to the effect that the child could not be kept in her special class, owing to the serious degree of her intellectual deficit and her instability of character.

The medical file was a collection prized by the father. He had organized it himself. He was careful to carry only copies of the medical certificates, keeping the originals at home in a safe where, as he put it, he had his other business papers. He was referring to files relating to his lawsuits against various members of his family. The father reminded me of a disjointed puppet. His voice was rasping and hoarse, his gestures overemphatic. His appearance was unkempt, his clothes stained, buttons missing, tie askew. He had the air of making me a present of his daughter. "She is something very special, like Aunt Eugenie [she was a schizophrenic aunt to whom we shall return later], but, in my opinion, she has something extra, some little perversion, quite slight, but still it shows."—"I've thought of being psychoanalyzed myself; it interests me. I've read Freud, I've got sexual obsessions, I could make an interesting case to you, but since Mireille is ill, it's enough to have one of us under analysis." It was in the same words that the mother was to tell me at the end of the treatment that it was enough to have one child in analysis, implying that at least one madman be left at large.

While the father was talking, the mother sat impassively, motionlessly, her hands crossed. Her skirt came down to her ankles. Her face was at once stern and childlike, her hair was forced back into a tight bun. The glasses she wore gave her the appearance of an aging, scared teenager. She obviously disapproved of her husband's remarks. Mireille suited her just as she was. The mother was afraid of being parted from her child. "When Mireille's around, I'm not frightened," she said. "We're trying psychoanalysis only to get her back into a special school," the father added.

The mother confessed hesitantly in the course of the interview that she had been depressed during pregnancy. "I don't know how

I got pregnant. It must have been from bathing in the sea." The baby had given her a lot of trouble. From her birth, Mireille had suffered from vomiting, anorexia, and at a later stage, insomnia. These facts were unmentioned during previous inquiries. (They were revealed to me after the mother had admitted to depression during pregnancy. I was to learn later that she had been subject to bouts of depression ever since the age of twelve.)

The father laughingly explained that he used to deal with Mireille's insomnia by forcing water into her to stop her crying. The couple made me feel uncomfortable. The child, whom I had not yet met, appeared through the speech of the parents as an instrument to serve the pleasure of one, and an object to soothe the anxiety of the other.

I interviewed Mireille a few days later. Cute, mischievous, pretty, with round cheeks, black eyes, and long tangled hair, the child looked like a little imp. Completely at ease, she ignored me, going from one toy to another, then sat down and started to draw. I explained to her that she was coming to tell me about the real things she felt, which sometimes scared her. The child began to speak and I was engulfed in words; they came and went, they danced up and down, and all the while she was busy drawing and modeling with clay. The words seemed to come from outside, they were being transmitted through her.

"Mireille, who's she?" was the question she asked at the first session. She did not expect a reply. Was it Mireille herself, or someone who asked the question through her?—that was my reaction. I did not start a conversation. Mireille was absorbed in making little objects. "They go into people's tummies and kill them."

"Into whose tummies?" I asked. "Do they really kill or make-believe kill?"

The child got up and started to march around, waving her arms in rhythm to the following incantation: "The parson's daughter speaks badly and doesn't know her name. The parson's father doesn't know his name, and the parson doesn't, either. Mireille talks to the parson and the parson's father, but they won't listen to her. They don't know what they're doing, they don't know who they are. Then Mireille gets fed up and takes a gun to shoot the parson and the grandfather. When they're dead, she eats them up."

The speech was in intent an accusation, but all association of ideas was rejected. The child sat down again and became absorbed in the same small objects. I was struck by the words which seemed to have come from outside and which hovered like riddles. My ears were still ringing with the father's accusations against his own father and brothers, and his wife's father and brothers. "I'll get even with the lot of them," he had said. And in fact it was *the character of* a Father that the child had introduced into a situation of mirror-aggression.

"Life for the little girl can't be easy in a family like that," I said to her.

The child strung together another speech, which also revolved in a vacuum: "When the little girl finishes eating the grandfather, her face gets all different and turns into a face without a name. In the face without a name there aren't any eyes, and there isn't any mouth, there are only big teeth. The little girl goes near the water and then she runs away. She is afraid of the big teeth and the face without a name. She can see herself in the water without eyes. So she runs off, a long, long way. Because it's awful to be watched with no eyes. She finds a pond. But she still keeps on seeing the same face without any eyes, and she can't talk any more, so she drowns herself."

For three months, the child talked on a series of subjects in which the themes of the Name of the Father, death, hate, and punishment recurred. My sole comment was, "It's not a very easy life for a little girl."

Mireille did not want me to talk; any attempt at symbolization aroused her anxiety. In three months' time the little girl learned to read with her mother. She proved capable of adapting to group activities in a special environment. Her speed in learning to read amazed us. Analysis enabled her not to be any longer in the place of an Other reading for her; now it was she herself who laughed, cried, and got angry with the characters in books.

The mother became depressed because she felt that Mireille was escaping from her. The father became impotent and threatened divorce. "I've had enough of my wife's play-acting. She's a hysteric, the doctor told me so. She wants to be made love to, then she changes her mind, she screams, she cries, or she runs away. I never know what to expect before, during, or after intercourse. And to think that Mireille has witnessed all this from the day she was born!"

"From the day she was born?"

"She slept in our room until her sister Carole was born. After that she was put in another room, and that's when she started to call out at night and get scared."

The father tried to join in the treatment on the same terms as the child; he elaborated on his grievances about his superiors at work, making use of her as well as of myself. "See what you're doing to me!" the mother seemed to be saying to me, and "Look how they're trying to hurt me," the father implied.

In dealing with Mireille's position in the family I came up against the attitude of the parents, which was conveyed to me in the disguise of the symptom. "My blood pressure is very high, I can't take my daughter to you," the mother would say. "My boss doesn't like the idea of my daughter's treatment. He's trying to block my promotion," the father would declare. Each of them, behind the mask, made clear the demand, the insistence that nothing be changed, as if the game could not continue under altered circumstances. Mireille knew what was at stake, since she repeated a phrase that clearly came from the mother: "Psychotherapy isn't for delicate children."

"That's what Mummy thinks," I replied. "You're her plug with your illness.[1] When you are not ill, it's Mummy who suffers from fears and fatigue. Your parents understand that we should continue psychotherapy."

The child looked at me for the first time, was silent for a moment, then roared with laughter. "Madame M. is in psychotherapy, but watch out, it makes you delicate."

Mireille got up, moved around, went to the window, and in a solemn voice declaimed: "In life, a man journeys down the road, leaves tracks, and then, poof, he disappears. Another man comes, leaves tracks, poof, he disappears. The third man comes and leaves tracks, but the thunder roars at everything that can't be blotted out."

"What are the tracks?"

"You know what they are. They are graves. There are lots and lots of them."

"The tracks are everything that can't be blotted out in the life of a little girl, and in the lives of the parents of the little girl, and the parents of the parents of the little girl. That's what Madame M. and Mireille are going to try to understand."

"There's nothing to understand. There isn't any God, and the thunder doesn't talk any more. It's said all it's got to say and now you're boring me."

"There's nothing to understand" was already the result of a structuring in analysis. The child reached it by a refusal, and immediately reverted to the type of communication in which she was spoken through. She was arrested at that point month after month. The *I* vanished, the name disappeared. The child insisted on being called Carole (the name of the younger sister to whom she was much attached), and clung to the phobic object as if to safeguard herself against the danger of any relation to desire. Her fear of sunlight and of noise put her into such a state of agitation that her parents suspended treatment, which happened the day Mireille, in a

---

[1] This term is employed to echo the manner in which the child situated herself as object in the place of the mother.

single outcry rediscovered *I*, in order to say, "I don't want to come
back any more."

"Mireille's place is with her brothers and sisters," the mother
wrote to me. "Psychotherapy is doing her harm." One could sense a
note of triumph in her lines; the mother had won, she had succeeded in keeping the child for herself.

Six months went by and a total of eighteen months had passed
since the first interview.

The father came to see me and related a dream: "My mother
gave me a job to do. I fell into a ravine. I was frightened and my
legs were cut off. I had to talk to a psychoanalyst about this dream.
I've brought Mireille back to you. I want you to give me some
protection against my wife."

It was because the father was subject to premature ejaculation
that he took it upon himself to bring his daughter back, while
handing me the task of protecting him against his wife. She did, in
fact, wield the authority, as he played being the boss—just as he
had played being his mother's husband when he was a child.

"Give me the name of an analyst," he asked, "I must go into
analysis myself."

I gave him a name; he never used it.

Mireille appeared and stood still between the double doors, in
territory that was neither inside my office nor outside it. "I don't
want to come in," she said.

"The last time you said 'I don't want to come back,' now you say
'I don't want to come in.' Why are you standing between the doors
even though you want something? If you come in, you will be with
me and we can perhaps figure out what it all means."

"No, no, no!" Mireille stamped her foot. She was holding a copy
of *Vogue* in one hand. She read anything, illustrated magazines,
children's books, *Elle, Paris-Match,* or *France-soir.* She carried
some reading matter with her wherever she went, anything would

do. However, she was incapable of telling about what she just read. Even phrases that registered came back distorted in some way. Some story from the Bible would merge with the White Witch and a news item to make up her context.

Mireille went on shouting. I began writing, taking no notice of her presence in the neutral territory. After a while I called out: "When there is a Father to give orders to Mummy and the little girl, it's much easier. The little girl needn't be afraid then. She knows where she is."

The child dropped the magazine, shut the doors, and came in. She stood motionless in front of me.

"Have you a lot of things to tell me?"

"Yes." The child lay down on the couch. When she spoke, it was the *I* of her mother that came through. "I've got a bad leg, it's breaking. I don't want to be a little woman, but a middle-sized woman. I'm afraid of being a little woman because that means I'm a little girl. I don't want to be a ridiculous woman. I'm not weak. But if you become a woman too soon, it makes you weak. It's a bad habit. Making love makes you weak. It's vulgar. You've got to be a real woman."

The father was suffering from impotence or premature ejaculation. The mother signified in her attacks that she was unable to accept her own lack. Mireille used her mother's words in her return. She was reflected as in a mirror. Although she introduced the phallic signifier, she was touching on the recognition points that caused the sinking of her parents; therefore, there seemed to be no solution for her other than to resume her role as the artificial support of her mother. In this way, each becomes the other's hostage. "When Mireille is with me, I'm not frightened of cars," says the mother. "Mummy wants Mireille to be like this, so why change?" replies the child.

Who regulates the therapy in psychoanalysis? The mother, the child, the father, or the analyst? Who wants the cure? What does getting well signify to the person who wants it? Why is Mireille here? In whose behalf? These were the questions that were to reveal their answers step by step in the course of treatment.

Mireille now appeared in her symptom as subject. She made her madness and stupidity the stakes in the analysis. She assumed the part of clown, she acted mad to entertain. Two new characters made their appearance at this time. One was a retarded cousin also named Mireille, the favorite of the paternal grandmother. (The two children had lived together between the ages of three and four.) The other was Aunt Eugenie, a schizophrenic aunt (actually, a distant cousin), the only person the father loved, with whom the child frequently stayed. Mireille delivered a succession of discourses. The word that revolved was that of the Other. Sustained by her own questioning, she was unable to introduce any symbolization of the desire of the Other. Since the Name of the Father had not worked, there was no axis around which her words could revolve. Who was talking through her? Was it Aunt Eugenie?

"Love, hot blood, long live the whores! Whores kiss and end up in the garbage can. A great night and all the poodles have puppies. The day said: I want the moon. Big Eva died raped."

The tale she was spinning amused her; she found Aunt Eugenie again in her clowning, and suppressed me. At other times, she was the speaking reflection of her mother; she borrowed her voice, her walk, her gestures, and smirking and prissy she writhed in front of the mirror, arranged an imaginary bun of hair and said: "Mireille is smarter than Mummy. Loza people get tumbled in bed. Loza girl screams. Loza boy says, shut up, I'm laying you." [2]

Was this a reference to something she had overheard? Several times she implied by various allusions (as had her father) that the real actress was Mummy, and that she, Mireille, knew a thing or two about their sexual bouts.

The child was held back in her progress by the unconscious wish

---

[2] Schizophrenic plays on words are, of course, untranslatable. The word "loza" is a reference to the part of France from which the family had come. (Translator's note.)

of the mother that nothing change. Mireille was doing so well in her special school that her teacher counseled a change in her educational environment and recommended sending her to boarding school. I encouraged the parents in this direction. Continuation of treatment thus led to a new phase—we were now aiming at something other than the initial wish of the family. A small boarding school for normal children was able to accept Mireille, and it was decided she should go. This coincided with the end of the second year of treatment. The mother was uneasy; she was not disposed to accept her husband's decisions, but she did not dare to oppose them openly. At the time of departure, the child seemed to be running a temperature, but the father said to her, "It's nothing. They've got everything they need to look after you at school." The little girl left without a scene. By using his daughter, the father succeeded in gaining the upper hand with his wife, but not for long. That night a doctor was summoned urgently. "Doctor," said the mother, "I'm dying. I'm hollow inside. I don't feel anything any more." Mireille, who used to fill that hollow, was indeed gone. Since the child was not available to prevail upon the father with an illness, the mother now set herself to the task by means of her symptom.

Away from her family, the child allowed herself desires and expressed demands (she wanted a doll, candy, money, and to learn dancing). A junior teacher would bring her to her sessions with me, but soon the father intervened. He would fetch Mireille from school and bring her, to the detriment of his work. His wife asked him to tell me that their other children missed Mireille. "What do you expect? It's only natural, isn't it? Mireille belongs to us," the father commented. The father's authority was sham, not real, and the child was aware of the deception. It was her mother who held the strings and pulled them. We were in a situation where each person was at once actor and victim in his chosen part.

More than two years passed. The first phase of the treatment was drawing to a close. By asking on the first day, "Mireille, who's she?" the child entered treatment, hidden behind stories that were posed as riddles. Her themes had developed from the absence of a surname for a Father, made a detour through a succession of small objects introjected as signifiers, and finally stressed the role played by the child as artificial support to her mother. She could not put her question without causing physical exhaustion in the mother and anxiety in the father. Mireille then gave up questioning and clung to her phobic object, namely, attacks of phobic anxiety or the role of the crazy girl, used as defense, against the anxiety of being torn from her identification with her parents. Mireille chose to be the symptom of one in a situation of complicity. "There are things the little girl doesn't want to see," she said to me, and then added, "When you're bored, you get sad and then you think that something is missing, that you're abandoned. When Mummy is sad she misses having children, she always wants others to be born so that she can feel full, instead of empty and lacking. To be without children makes her unhappy."

Mireille was not able to touch upon the castration problem without involving the respective positions of her parents in relation to the signifier (phallus, the Name of the Father), which would have provoked their collapse.

"Mireille is living the life of a lady," said the father, "she hit the jackpot, but things can't go on like this." The child was taken out of school and returned to the pathogenic home environment. In her quest for a solution, she chose to continue in her role as being mad. "The sun could make the little girl better, but he destroys her for fun. Nothing can be done." The child defined here the limits of therapeutic action. What was being destroyed? On this point, Mireille remained silent; it was for me to comprehend. In the vacuum from where Mireille was seeing me, words had no meaning. She clearly defined herself as a girl as opposed to a boy, contrasted life with death, introduced the idea of parenthood and the prohibition of incest; the major themes appeared, filling in meanings that had been lost, but there was no central axis. Not only did it seem impossible to grasp a Symbolic order, but if anything on this level seemed obtainable, the father intervened at precisely that moment in reality to destroy it. He admitted to me that he examined the child's sexual parts, took her temperature, and watched for signs of puberty. "On the trains, in the streets, I always have the feeling that all men have eyes only for her and want to be up to their dirty tricks."

"Prisons and daddies are like that," echoed the child, "God should not make things like that."

As details were gradually filled in about the father, so the child signified the impossibility of getting better while the adults remained mad. "Mummy and Daddy don't want any more psychotherapy for Whore. They accept it only with certain conditions. And for Whore, God is one huge psychotherapy."

The theme of God was to recur at the end of the treatment in a dream, in which Mireille, as a boy, was summoned by God, that is, summoned to die.

"What I say cuts no ice with Mireille," the father said to me. "I'm annoyed with her. She doesn't believe me, and the worst of it is that she's quite right. My authority is slipping. I think she's improved enough. After all, she's got to adjust to her family, not to society. What is society? Nothing but venality and treachery—everything's rotten."

I replied, "It isn't easy for Mireille to get better when she's not the only one involved."

The father visibly sank. "It's quite true," he said, "we need Mireille as she is."

A few days later, he had a paranoiac delirium. The child was injured in a car accident and witnessed a brawl in which her father injured an opponent.

"The men in my family," said the child, "they are all of them rude words which I won't say. Psychotherapy came along and the little girl became her own self." Then she added "No, I can't do that to her. I want to be where I ought to be, near Mummy."

After this avowal, Mireille reverted to her initial prophetic style, conjuring up a succession of myths from beyond herself. I was moved by these myths, produced at a time when the child was witness to the disordered behavior of a paranoiac father. I perceived their message as the echo of the impossible situation that had been created for her. It was from that base that the child introduced the idea of God while continuing to imply the namelessness of the father. As for the father, filled as he was with hate for his own father, he was engaged in legal proceedings about legacies, not only with his own three brothers but also with the men in his wife's family. In response to the real risk of death to which she had been exposed with her father, Mireille conjured up the myth of the three great kings and the myth of the three men. *The three great kings* crossed Mireille's path to show her the place of good and evil. One of the kings said she had sinned and she drowned herself.

In the myth of *the three men,* the child told the following story: "A man looked after you. He was old, fifty-seven years old. You are thirty-nine. You are married. You say to yourself: Iron man, black iron man who makes wooden shoes, here they are then. You can choose between a white man and a black man. You chose the one who was your father's man and brought him wooden shoes. Your man was made of iron. He made iron clogs. He was thinking about your father. Your father slapped the iron man, who cried. He was your husband. Then you chose another man who pleased your father better; he was the hairdresser's man. Your father was getting old. You left three men. Then you had black men to play with until you had enough of them. You gave them to your cousin on your wedding day. The iron man and the black man got drunk. You finished your life with a man and you obeyed him."

Drama was smoldering in Mireille's family. Every time the child seemed to get herself launched, she experienced a mutilation in reality which overwhelmed her.

The father's mother died. The father wanted to assume the mourning as his own private task, not to be shared. A row broke out with the third brother, whom he accused of murder. Through the mirror-play in which he was imprisoned he revealed what he wanted to be: "I must become an honest robber or a fine murderer." Something got trapped and could no longer be expressed. Mireille then took over the role and played the king's jester. She told the truth concerning Father. "It isn't Daddy who's in charge. Daddy acts mad. He is mad. But it's a secret. Daddy plays mean tricks on himself. He does things daddies shouldn't do. The Lord arrived too late to help me."

The child was to make no further progress. She had already told me what she had to tell. Firmly imprisoned in her symptom, she refused to be dislodged from her position by an interpretation. For a long time, she had an option: madness or cure, life or death, either for herself or for her parents. In this choice, Mireille was referring us to her father's madness. She could face it only by wearing the mask of one retarded or mad. To the last, the child sought to fill in lost meanings; she rehabilitated the memory of her paternal grandfather through the picture of the good grandmother: "She was old, Daddy's mummy. She used to tell me stories about a man she liked a lot. She had a good time with him."

Whenever Mireille tried to gain some measure of control in her words, she came up against some dimensions in the parents which could not be mentioned without provoking their collapse.

"It's with you that I'm crazy," Mireille said one day, "not with the others." Then she explained the advantage of her symptom: "What makes the crazy girl happy is that people laugh at her."

At the same juncture, the child asked her mother: "If people who are abnormal do it on purpose, is it all right?"

Whether madness or retardation, Mireille seemed to regard it as an illness to be developed for the Other or with the Other, thereby implying that she was the subject in it. And so Mireille brought me her last story and left me her disguise: "It isn't me speaking, it's my disguise," she said.

One might ask whether the child was not speaking from the

locus I was situated in as she put the story into words; the disguise used here consists of the word of Madame M. *plus* Mireille. "You can't be well. You can't tell the difference between the you and the I, so you must be crazy. What makes me laugh is that there is someone who has mixed up Madame M. and Madame M. It's good to mix things up. It's life. It's very nice to mix up laughter and crying and the law of God. Life is monstrous; you are monstrous. You are one of the monsters. You didn't trust anyone; you only got your word to help you. And it helped you to die. The word of others wasn't rich enough. Your difficulty stopped you from listening to them. The others listened to your word, but they didn't do anything good with it. You were quite wrong about eternal life and about the life of the kings. In the end, your word wasn't listened to. The rest was for you, but you didn't do anything with it. You weren't capable of doing anything with it. The iron man smashes your lungs into little pieces because he is feeling bad. He really does hurt people. So what? That's life."

A few days earlier, in connection with telling a story in which "a father burgled his daughter," the child said, "When a daughter replaces the wife for her father, she dies of it."

After this story, the tone of her discourse changed and she became reserved in expressing herself. She depicted members of her family with ferocity. She drew up a balance sheet: Why did she have a mad father, a useless mother, one brother who couldn't read, another who had enuresis, and a maid who was illiterate? Was it possible that all this was the will of God? Then she related a dream: "There was a boy dying, summoned by God. That boy is me. I don't want to die. Things are going well at school but counting is still difficult. If God doesn't exist, I wish he did somewhere all the same."

Counting for an Other. Counting also appeared to be the fulcrum of the father's delusions: "If it isn't me they want to get rid of, who is it? There are four of us and the inheritance was split three ways."

Mireille started treatment by posing the myth of the three men through the voice of thunder roaring at everything that could not be blotted out. We find the same myth at the end, referring us to the delusions of the father and to his perverted relationship with his daughter. It is at this level that Mireille remained trapped.

Was Mireille mentally retarded or psychotic? This was the question I asked myself after four years of psychoanalysis.

I was struck from the outset by the astonishing richness of words conjured up by Mireille from beyond herself, manifesting a truth that indited parents, grandparents, and great-grandparents. Where do the words, the rhythm, the poetry come from in these children who are overwhelmed too young by an incomprehensible drama? Guy also used a certain type of discourse which contrasted in its richness with his otherwise poor power of communication.

> Daddy committed many sins
> Before his death he was quite worn out.
> He was so weary,
> It went on far too long.
> He was crushed and he died.
> He blew up and he died.
> So peace was restored at last.

His paranoiac father had committed suicide and the child was not deemed fit to know. The unsaid in these cases always assumes exceptional importance. It generally refers to what the child knows, but does not want to know.

Treatment by psychoanalysis might save such children from psychiatric commitment, but it cannot always preserve the promise they seem to have in them; as it progresses, their discourse gradually loses color, and the child is "adjusted"—at what cost? Sometimes, at the cost of destroying a certain form of self-fulfillment. If the child sustains physical damage (through illness or accident), he is apparently more likely to retain the verbal richness which others lose as they get better. (Such loss coincides with the subsiding of substitute phenomena, when all possibility of symbolization has failed. The loss also occurs in cases where the patient, owing to the way treatment develops, approaches the stance of the neurotic, introducing defense mechanisms against the return of repressed materials.)

In order to clarify what is involved, let us restate it. Such children were prematurely injured, perverted, or thwarted in the locus of their desire. Since the oral stage, their need has brought death, as the mother's demand was to keep the baby from awakening to desire. Crippled in the representation he is able to form of his body, such a child is further weighed down by the denial of his genitals, the seat of desire. He is disoriented in relation to the primal scene, because he encounters nothing but fantasies and death-wishes at the parental level. The task of analysis is to contrive to resurrect the child from this early death. It is not always possible. The prognosis for a cure depends partly on the strength of the link between the child and the pathogenic parent. The case of Mireille raises in a particularly acute form a problem commonly encountered in child psychoanalysis. The analyst finds himself confronted from the outset with the impotence, perversion, criminality, or madness of an adult whose words are disseminated through the family. The child makes himself the embodiment of a curse or, more simply, of the unrevealable. Two forms of discourse are available to him: direct communication, which is often very poor, or the speech of tragedy or farce transmitted through him. In the latter, he succeeds at a certain juncture in situating himself as subject, in order to conserve a language of myth and story which serves him to express the inexpressible.

As previously unsayable things gradually come to be said, the child abandons myths and reverts to direct speech, apparently with the choice of remaining prisoner in a certain verbal poverty, or of overcoming it by acquiring access as subject to the world of symbols where words convey meaning. It is only then that the child has resolved his problem analytically. This stage is not easy to attain and the risk of an impasse persists to the end.

. . .

Here we touch on the problem of the limitations of analysis from the technical point of view. *For whom must the child continue to be mad when he is no longer mad?* This is the question. My position is to undertake treatment even in hopeless cases, if I get a certain measure of consent from the parents and if they accept the dialogue. The most pessimistic prognosis is disproved as regularly as the most optimistic one. The types of discourse I have recorded in certain cases are so astonishing that I have been accused of inducing, even inventing them. There is a problem here which might deserve closer examination. Because a child finds it possible to say what he feels to be *true* to a person to whom he attributes the power of not only knowing his thoughts but also of unmasking what remains unsaid, he can draw from another world—with incantations derived from others—what could not be conveyed in his own words any more than it could be in our own regular vocabulary. What is wrested from such children is the wrath of the poet or of the gods, and it is from this revolt that something can be eventually verbalized. The analyst gets a legend, one that the parents have enveloped it in.

Laurence, nine years old, stood petrified upon opening the door. Not a sound came from her mouth. She devoured me with her gaze, then threw herself into my arms and laid her head on my shoulder. I said nothing. I stroked her hair.

"Then it's true, you really are Madame M.?"

"Yes, I am. Can you tell me what Madame M. means for you?"

A long silence. "She's the person who doesn't muddle up names. It isn't nice to muddle up names."

Another pause. Then Laurence started a different type of communication, a schizophrenic one, which she was to sustain with me thereafter.

Such children scarcely need to have the purpose of analysis explained to them. One might say, in some cases, that they have been waiting for it all their lives. They have been waiting to meet someone who is designated—owing to his inner capacity to perceive the drama—to hear that which is beyond the range of words to be recognized by the Other.

Laurence was born after a stillborn brother, Laurent. She felt that her mother desired her to be dead. She knew nothing about the brother, yet this was the knowledge she offered me at the outset.

Mireille told me that there was nothing to understand: "The thunder doesn't talk any more. It's said all it's got to say and now you're boring me." Nevertheless, she went on talking, now rebelliously, now seriously—the words flowed on, and sometimes she was not in them and sometimes she was—what I mean is that she acquired access beyond herself to myths, to make intelligible the unbearable truth, the inhuman loneliness. And then, it became clear that the reign of the gods was over. The child who wished to remain detached began talking on another level about the problem that still remained, and that she could then tackle without a mask. The type of discourse the child employs from the outset of treatment continues because of another parallel development. The parents, in their turn, are also talking or not talking to the analyst about the child—that is, they are presenting their problem, or rather the fantasies the child has represented by his symptom.

The mother expressed her grievances through Mireille, the father his claims. The child's speech rhythms alternated with those of the parents. "It's like two sides of a magic box," the father observed in reply to one of my remarks. "When the red lights up on this side, the green lights up on the other." Mireille's evolution (her questioning of sex, death, the paternal metaphor) endangered first one, then the other parent. Each one intervened in his own way to stop the treatment or to circumscribe its effects. The mother clearly expressed her wish to "keep Mireille as she was." (We have seen that any separation induced phobic anxiety or somatic attack in her.) To hear the mother is not the same as analyzing her; inviting her to speak enabled her to verbalize what remained otherwise unsaid, and the unsaid included her sexual fantasies which the child represented in her symptom (her demeanor and speech as a mad child). Mireille's mission consisted in masking the sexual aberrations of her parents, and this brings us back to the Oedipal problem of the parents.

We have seen how the father's perverted relationship with his daughter made it impossible for her to repress her own Oedipal problem. Mireille seemed to have no meaning for him, unless she was seen in a certain context, through the keyhole of his voyeurism. The father was what he was—and I had no option but to listen to him. By way of Mireille, he conveyed to me his Oedipal problem, his hatred for his brothers, his sexual obsessions. His relationship with his child consisted of a succession of anal aggressions, car accidents exposing her to danger, and verbal threats of death. Mireille's sexual parts were spoken of and inspected, but the child had no right to have them for herself.

The mother was the passive accomplice of the father's assaults on the child. What they were both really seeking through their daughter, was a form of sexual gratification which presupposed, as far as the child was concerned, the obliteration of her sexual parts, which were not allowed to be her private property. When the parents said, "Mireille belongs to us," they were referring to her sexual parts as well as to herself as a "sick" child. Although she had not yet reached puberty, they were already preoccupied with the idea that she might not remain a virgin. When Mireille laid aside her mad style of speech at the end of treatment to relate her first dream, she revealed what she believed to be her mother's wish concerning her: ". . . to be a boy who is dying, summoned by God."

The impasse in Mireille's treatment is attributable to her never seeing any solution to the situation created for her, except death or non-desire. As subject of desire, Mireille was most of the time in a state of suspense, as strikingly manifested by the appearance and disappearance of the *I*. It was only in the context of her "illness" that she seemed to have the right to count at the level of desire (since she cancelled herself out of it). Mireille both disappeared into her "illness" and clung to it. She disappeared so that the dialogue with the Other might be conducted indirectly through her symptom. (It was her madness that concerned adults.) She clung to it, drawing from the Imaginary a reply that became a recognition point, even if it was an alibi. (In the transference situation, Mireille asked me to collaborate in her defense mechanism.) Throughout the treatment, the child was seeking in the speech of the Other a third element that might intervene to impose order, and release her from a dual situation that had no outlet. But she came up against the father's wish—"I must become an honest robber or a fine murderer"—implying "I intend to remain outside any Law, I who am a representative of the Law." [3] Bouts of violence in a father of potentially murderous power put Mireille into a state of confusion that she did not want to see. The father attracted her by his intelligence, although on another level he exposed her to danger. As for the mother, the child despised her in all fields. The child had no one she could count on; when she remarked at the end of treatment, ". . . counting is still difficult," she expressed the wish to situate somewhere a transcendental Father figure, in contrast to the real father for whom *counting* meant murder or suicide. Intuitively, the little girl knew the recognition points she needed, but she had great difficulty in working through her mourning for those that were lacking in her parents, particularly in her father. This is what brought about the impasse.

In her progress she shared the effects produced in the parents' unconscious. We can distinguish two phases here. In one, Mireille responded to the unconscious desire of her mother by becoming an object to mask the mother's anxiety. An illness was required for this, any would do. What mattered was to prevent the mother from becoming depressed by occupying her with cares and worries. On this level, one could say that Mireille embodied the symptom of her parents, of her mother in particular. Subsequently, through the

[3] The father was a high official in the police.

process of transference, I took over and shouldered parental anxiety. The child could then evolve in her own name, as it were. The second phase is situated at this juncture, but it is not always clearly distinguished from the first. Mireille appears in it as subject while continuing to be someone's symptom.

In the first phase, treatment was not conducted in her name. She was, in turn, Mireille + Madame M., Mireille + mother, Mireille + Aunt Eugenie, Mireille + cousin. I was her accomplice in what she was unwilling to see or hear; she made me collaborate in her defense mechanism, while on the other side of the transference situation she defended herself against the threat of being voyeuristically devoured. Mireille suppressed me in the role of the Other in her attacks of hypomania, and thereafter appeared only behind various masks. The *I* was eclipsed, the name was effaced. When Mireille appeared in her words behind the mask of Mireille + mother, it was to indicate in this capacity that the real actress was the Other and not herself. She was also heard through the words of Aunt Eugenie, the schizophrenic aunt her father was so fond of. She established herself as Mireille the fool, in the manner of the mentally retarded cousin of the same age and name, who was the favorite of her paternal grandmother. She took refuge in a series of identifications, even identifying with the father, whose words she occasionally assumed. The child seemed caught in a form of narcissism during these withdrawals, in order to protect herself from the anxiety of being torn from her identification with her parents. Mireille did not succeed in facing this, except through the circuit of myths she conjured up from within herself, in a hopeless quest for possible symbolization. It was at this point where she found herself forced back on her parents' own problem, where their speech superimposed itself, and where the game of decoy started between them and herself. Whenever the child seemed ready to get launched into a phase of progress, the father intervened in reality by a form of aggression, bringing her back to a field where any process of symbolization was doomed to failure. The child at that moment effaced herself in front of the signifier of "illness," and remained under the banner marked by the device of the Other.

At this juncture of the second phase she revealed the nature of her symptom. "If people who are abnormal do it on purpose, is it all right?" was the question she asked her mother, while to me she confessed, "It's with you that I'm crazy, not with the others." She meant that people were mad for the Other and with the Other, and that, by Heaven, she was ready to accept me in the part. I thus became the person for whom she maintained her symptom. Although Mireille had recovered a normal intelligence[4] and satisfactorily adjusted to schooling, and although her language had become coherent, analytically speaking, she could still not be regarded as cured. It was always possible that she would have recourse to other symptoms for someone else.

The problem of castration was not brought up during treatment; whenever Mireille appeared to be raising the matter, questioning was directed through the parents and this brought persecutory reactions from them. Mireille, in fact, could not take a stand on the issue that her mother lacked a phallus, without causing her to disintegrate. When the child was carried away by her questioning, she was trying in vain to find a central axis around which to organize what she was saying. There was no taking hold of the Name of the Father, there was no reference possible to the mother, the child was in a vacuum. It was from the vacuum that she looked to me. If I gave a meaning to her words, she broke off her game, but she became anxious when a chance of symbolization arose. In the game of decoy she conducted with her parents or the analyst, there was no symbolization for the desire of the Other. It was her symptom of madness that she used as stake, and from it she took her flights into a series of identifications in which we see Mireille reflected infinitely.

[4] Her results in intelligence tests were uneven. She succeeded in tests of mathematical reasoning at the level of an average adult, but failed in an arithmetical problem for a nine-year-old. She also succeeded in tests of ingenuity for a fourteen-year-old while failing in a problem for an eight-year-old. She succeeded when she wanted to; the tests were a game in which she made her own rules.

．　．　．

We have encountered three types of discourse in Mireille. (i) The child was spoken through by her mother, Aunt Eugenie, her cousin, Madame M., and her father. (ii) When she spoke as subject, there was nothing, since nothing was at stake. She introduced the key words of the unsaid, the major words revolved, drowned in speech, but had no significant interrelationship. (iii) As a result of structuring in analysis, the presence of Mireille made itself felt, and the *I* first took on a meaning in the form of a negation—the "I don't want to come back" at the beginning of treatment, and the "I don't want to die" at the end. Between these two phases, the child conjured up myths, but the signifiers revolved in a vacuum: good, evil, birth, death, father, seemed as attempts at substituting for lost meanings. Mireille's effort to introduce the figure of the good grandmother, who used to tell her stories about a man, perhaps indicated a juncture when there was an attempt to structure hysteria as a defense against psychotic mechanisms.

In the analysis, transference occurred to the extent that something of the Symbolic order did get through to her, despite the anxiety that any symbolization caused her.

Was Mireille mentally retarded or psychotic? That was the question at the beginning of treatment. At the end of it, I wondered whether analysis had not made her into a hysteric at one point, who identified with the psychotic aunt. I now put the question whether psychosis sprang up because at a given moment hysteria failed to establish itself as a defense mechanism. The diagnoses of retardation and psychosis were made at precisely the time when the child was in difficulty about her recognition points. The exceptionally long treatment resulted from the special relationship of the child with a paranoiac and perverted father, and a hysterical and "delicate" mother. (This, incidentally, raises the complex problem of the limitations of analysis with children brought up in very disturbed homes.) To conclude, let us listen to Mireille's mother: "At the age of seven, Jacques is now saying all the disgusting, senseless, and vulgar things Mireille used to say. He has no restraint any more. I really ought to bring him to you, but it's enough to have had one child in psychoanalysis, I won't give you another." When Mireille was no longer in the special place that concealed the mother's own anxiety from herself, was Jacques coming into the game, or rather, into the net spread by the mother for the satisfaction of her own needs? This was the question I was asking myself when Mireille let drop these words in one of the last sessions: "My difficulty is that I always have to have someone to speak through." She did not necessarily mean a real person. The recognition of what she called her "difficulty" in effect indicated an impasse. She had continually taken me back to this point throughout the treatment, thereby designating the field where she had lost, hidden, or disguised herself.

CHAPTER VIII

CONCLUSIONS

In his preface to Aichhorn's *Wayward Youth*[1] Freud admitted that psychoanalytic research had shifted from the study of neurotics to the study of children. He added the observation: "Analysis has shown how the child lives on unchanged in the sick man as well as in the dreamer and the artist."

Child psychoanalysis proposes an approach that does not differ essentially from that in the analysis of neurotic adults. All questions asked in analysis come from an Other, and are about the other in the patient.[2] The analysand constitutes himself as the speaking subject, starting from the feeling that he is addressing someone bearing the imprint of an experience common to them both. This relationship of trust is based on the model of that earliest relationship which links the child to his mother. It is as subject contemplated by the Other that the analysand initially constitutes himself as speaking subject, and the failure of the relationship is linked to that which went wrong in the mother-child dialectics, it

---

[1] S. Freud, "Preface to Aichhorn's *Wayward Youth*," Standard Edition, Vol. XIX, p. 273.

[2] J. Lacan, "Les Formations de l'inconscient," *Bulletin de psychologie*, Vol. XII, Nos. 2–4 (November–December, 1958).

arising again in the type of discourse being articulated in the analysis.

The play between mother and child is established as soon as the child makes a demand, and if the mother's response creates a feeling in the child that he is rejected as subject of desire, he will remain identified with the partial object which is the object of his mother's demand, without ever being able to progress further, or to assume words of his own. We can situate the nexus of psychotic conditions in this. In cases where some analysts talk about environment, surroundings, and behavior, we must respond by analyzing the type of discourse used by the parents in front of (or to) the child. The possibility of treatment lies in our understanding the characteristics of the adults' words that have left their imprint on the child. In a psychoanalytic case history, it is not so much the correctly ordered facts that count, as the meaning that can be given to them as they are put into play through the message given to the analyst. We are faced with the effects of what has been said to the child, or passed over in silence. It is impossible to approach psychosis so long as the psychotic remains another stranger to himself for the analyst (i.e., so long as the analyst's resistance is reinforced by the fact that the psychotic is the Other and not the analyst). By returning the interrogation of the unanalyzable in the psychosis to the analyst[3] and no longer leaving it to the patient, the analytic situation is made possible.

In child psychoanalysis, we must also first ask ourselves questions about that other within ourselves, that is to say, we must contrive to find out what defines our position in relation to the child we are treating. By listening to what the child and his parents say to us, we are enabled to orient ourselves in relation to their discourse, and to discover with whom we are being identified.

Any analytic approach includes transference, the patient's as well as the analyst's, which involves bringing a complex interplay of

[3] P. Aulagnier, "Essai d'approche d'une conception psychanalytique des psychoses" (unpublished).

identifications to the surface. If the analyst fails to recognize this necessity, he runs the risk of treating the child as an absolute other, in order to get rid of that other within himself by means of projection or repression. In this way, the patient is transformed into an alien object in whose behalf measures can be taken, instead of efforts made to give meaning to the disorder in which he is alienated. *Attempts are made to provide better surroundings without reflecting on the fact that the surroundings consist, above all, in the collective discourse in which the subject is trapped.*

Studying the mechanism of identification does not mean that the analyst defines himself as father, mother, or child, for such terms can prove to be interchangeable. The point is that the analyst must admit what is in play for him in a given situation, which means that he must define the relation linking him to his own desire. What is thus in play in a relationship situation is the relation of each participant to the object of his desire, from the baseline of what he imagines to be the relation of the Other to himself as object of desire.

When the mother *demands* of her child that he should be clean, the child "gives" her his excrements and *identifies* them as the object of the demand, but the mother's demand (obedience) is in effect aimed at the *subject*. She is seeking in him something of the order of her own desire, and she will identify the object of her demand with the object of her desire.[4] The question that will sustain the child is, "What does my mother want?" We know that he will not find the answer until he has been able to interpose in his relationship with his mother something of the order of the Law (which presupposes the overcoming of the castration complex). So long as he does not succeed in doing this, he will remain wavering in an identification conflict.

What we see at the so-called pregenital stage is the manner in which the subject interiorizes one type of relation to the partial object by way of designating himself to the Other as object of de-

[4] Developed by P. Aulagnier, "Sur le concept d'identification (unpublished).

195

sire. It is precisely that—his manner of designating himself as object of desire—which we must grasp in his message. In a descriptive fashion, we might say that the superego of one is being identified with the superego of the other, but this is not the point that interests me. I have tried to steer clear of categorizing descriptions throughout this book in favor of the dynamics in play in a situation. Melanie Klein set the example for this approach by always talking about positions and situations, not stages of development. She was, however, always careful to provide the possibility for controlled experiment. She endeavored to place her clinical discoveries in a context that took into consideration the "affective development" of the individual. This book has a more limited scope; my concern has been to give an account of the analytic drama, and to show that it can be pinpointed only by means of a technique linked to a certain conception of analysis. In matters ascribed by the behaviorists to the influence of environment, we detect the effects of words that have been heard, whether understood or not, which form another sort of impalpable environment in a perspective that is no longer a biological one. I listen to a vast discourse, not only that of the child and his family, but also that of the past from which one can learn or reconstruct the words the child had lived with previously.

I have tried to show in this book why parents must bring their words to their child's analyst, and I have opposed the conception of psychoanalysis as "corrective experience" that can be continued by the mother at home. I have given some indication of how misleading that view is. The analyst who treats families with that method never inquires into the place of the mother's words in the fantasy world of the child, or the place of the father in the mother's words. He listens to the facts in their reality, but lets the meaning escape him. It is accepted that a given father is "bad," without going into what underlies the mother's complaint, and without asking what advantages she derives from the situation she has chosen to describe. By studying the child as a phenomenon, the analyst deprives himself of the requisite assistance of the parents' words; when he does invite the parents to speak, it is by way of getting information about the child's upbringing. There seems to be little concern about what is in play in the fantasy of the parents' desire. In obliging parents to enter analysis themselves, the analyst fails to see that it is useless to analyze a mother for her own sake when her own sake is the child to such an extent that she expresses her presence through the child's symptom (a symptom that bears the imprint of her desire). I have shown how the separate analysis of mother and child leaves untilled the entire field where the words of the child *and* the mother are constituted. The analyst himself is present in such symptomatic words in the home, but if he does not listen to the mother, he cannot determine what place he occupies in her fantasy. Also, as a result of not having been listened to by her child's analyst, the mother is likely to remain hidden behind the structure of her defenses. It is true that what the mother *says* will manifest itself through the child's words, but in such cases improvement in the child creates serious somatic or psychological attacks in the pathogenic parent. And, in the end, the symptom persists because the analyst has made himself the unwitting accomplice in the deceiving word. Belief in a positive explanation contrives in all these cases to hamper the progress of treatment. I have pointed out repeatedly the need for detecting what the child represents in the fantasy world of the parents (and of the analyst), because the child is not only the object of all their projections but also, more importantly, serves to mask the adult's lack of being. I have tried to show also that meaning appears in an analysis only by situating the subject more accurately in his words in relation to his demand and his desire.

My approach has nothing in common with one generally referred to as "family psychotherapy." [5] Adherents to this school are in opposition to "missionary" analysts who believe in helping disturbed children by "killing" their mothers (they are nicknamed

[5] Nathan W. Ackerman, "Family Psychotherapy," *American Journal of Psychotherapy,* Vol. XX, No. 3, (July, 1966).

"mother killers"). The family psychotherapists want to "save the family to save the child," but their methods have their source in the same missionary spirit. They counsel, they rehabilitate, they offer therapy as an orthopedic expedient. In comparing the analysis of a neurotic to a sort of "post-education," Freud made it very clear that it has nothing to do with any form of rehabilitation or pedagogy. What matters only is the effect of analysis on the patient's ability to respond in his own name to "moral education."

We listen to the parents' discourse because it explains what is nameless in the child. Divergences between the words of one parent and the other may sometimes account for a misunderstanding. (It may be useful to study its meaning subsequently with the child.) Erik Erikson is masterful at making use of the unsaid that surfaces during the child's treatment.[6] (The unsaid appears to be particularly important in traumatic neuroses.) Erikson's difficulties start, as we have seen, when he tackles the problem of psychoses; here he departs from the study of language and relies on a theory of development that makes it impossible for him to grasp what is really at issue in treatment.

My goal is to seek out and pin down a *message*. I stop at the subject who *is missing* in the diagnosis, after and beyond a nosological description. His place must be pinpointed in the vast expanse of words involving child, parents, and analyst. My opinions on this point are akin to those expressed by Laing and Esterson,[7] although Laing based his studies on patients he did not follow up in treatment, whereas I have endeavored to link my researches closely to the actual progress of my treatments. My point of reference was to

[6] Erikson, *Childhood and Society*.

[7] "We reiterate that we ourselves are not using the term *schizophrenia* to denote any identifiable condition that we believe exists 'in' one person. However, insofar as the term summarizes a set of clinical attributions made by certain persons about the experience and behavior of certain others, we retain the term for this set of attributions. We put in parentheses any judgment as to the validity or implications of such a set of attributions" (*Sanity, Madness and the Family*). These authors, however, adopt a different (phenomenological or existential) perspective.

seek out the enigma of the symptom by paying attention to the words of *child and parents* regarded as an entity.

My method is linked to the effects of tensions, compromises, misunderstandings, etc., in the discourse, the meaning of which in each individual history can be clarified by reference to the Oedipal drama or the castration experience. The uncovering of the meaning springs from a conflict situation (support of contradictory desires). The child responds by his symptom to that which has been cancelled out or destroyed in a fragment of the adult's speech. His words take shape in the locus of the Other and are linked with the fashion in which the relations of kinship, the metaphor of the father, etc., are structured in the other.[8] His accession as subject depends on the parents' desire to let him or not let him be born to the state of desiring. In the transference area, parents and child find themselves confronting at one point what they believe to be the analyst's desire.

The unfolding of a treatment involves bringing to light the factors in play in the experience of child-parent separation. The separation is lived with reference to the analyst through the death-wish, and it is then that child and parent assert themselves as each being the object lacking to the other. The analyst is called upon to choose the one he will agree to destroy. The child, in his attempts to establish himself as subject, encounters that element in his parents' unconscious which obstructs the accession of his being. In other words, he cannot engage in castration dialectics without challenging to some extent the parent to whom he is attached. The child's treatment touches on the adult's position in relation to desire.[9] The

---

[8] What the subject encounters is the signifier of the Other.

[9] "The important thing is to grasp where the organism is rooted in the subject's dialectics. This organ of the unreal in the living being is set by the subject at a given moment into the period when his separation takes place. It is actually his death that he makes the object of the Other's desire. All other objects that come in place of this will be substitutes borrowed from what he loses (excrement), or from what he finds in the Other which may serve as a prop of his desire—his look, his voice." J. Lacan, "Position de l'inconscient," *Écrits*, p. 829.

analyst must be able to situate himself in the discourse that is going on, so as to make dialectics possible. It is then that a true word will emerge from a death-wish. Then, out of death, division, and alienation, the subject will come into being in analysis, as a subject who speaks, which means one born of a drama that has marked and molded him.

Appendices

A CHALLENGE TO
MENTAL RETARDATION[1]

Freud Opens an Era

If we consult the past, we find that society entrusted to civil servants and jurists the task of drawing an acceptable boundary line
between sanity and insanity. Madness—like leprosy—was singled
out at a certain point in history, and subsequently defined by the
Church and jurisprudence. It appears to have been the jurist Zacchias[2] who gave such a subtle analysis of imbecility in the seventeenth century that it was later incorporated by the physician Esquirol in his classification of the mental debilities.

In the seventeenth century, there already existed an early model
of what was to evolve into our intelligence level tests. Categories
were drawn up according to the adaptability or social usefulness of
the mentally retarded. The objective was not so much to understand the mentally retarded person but to assign him a place, from
the juridical point of view, in a society primarily concerned with
safeguarding family property.

It was not possible to establish a proper human relationship with
one who was lunatic, simple-minded, or retarded. This failure was

---

[1] First appeared in a special number of *Esprit,* "L'Enfance handicapée" (November, 1965).

[2] Paul Zacchias, *Quaestiones medico-legales* (Lyons, 1674).

to become the source of the entire scientific rationale behind the disorders of insanity. The *truth* about madness and mental insufficiency came under study.

We owe the introduction of doctors into asylums to Tuke and Pinel, just at the time when these pioneers were coming to realize the non-medical role of the doctor and regard the doctor-patient relationship as the essential support of all therapy.[3] Still, the doctor made his appearance in the guise of judge, thus creating just another concentration camp for the insane. Although freed of their chains, they were subject to a moral judgment and were forced into another form of alienation of their being. "It is not so much a question of understanding madness," said the specialists of the day, "as of controlling it." (At that time, retardation and psychosis formed one nosologic entity.)

The realization of the doctor-patient link had to await Freud to acquire meaning and be put into practice; he made it possible to renew contact with sense on the far side of non-sense.

As a clinician, Freud was open to all discoveries; he mistrusted the propensity to classify and listened to the suffering that spoke in his patient. His stance was not taken up in relation to the truth of madness but in relation to a being endowed with the word who possessed a truth that was hidden from him, or eluded him, or was no longer his. A new era opened up for psychiatry, and the task of psychoanalysts above all is not to let the opening close down again. It might well be a cause of concern that the very success of psychoanalysis will in some measure arrest its progress as it inevitably becomes institutionalized. It is a fact that many psychoanalysts turn away from the problem of mental retardation and evade the exchange of ideas taking place on the subject. It took some time to admit psychosis into the analytic kingdom; even Freud believed that it was inaccessible to analysis. Little by little, in the wake of isolated and at first disputed successes, analysis has been proving itself as the best approach to schizophrenia. One might pose the

---

[3] Michel Foucault, *Madness and Civilization: A History of Insanity in the Age of Reason* (New York, Pantheon Books, 1965; London, Tavistock, 1967).

question of there being an analogous extension of psychoanalysis perhaps to certain cases of mental retardation.

The obstacles that distort communication between a normal person and a retarded one seem to be the same as the difficulties that had made the approach to psychosis impossible in the past. The negation, rejection, and objectification of the insane as subject of scientific study result from the "normal" person's failure to recognize not only his own fear but also his own sadistic daydreaming, and more importantly, the myths and superstitions that clouded his childhood and, unknown to himself, still live on in him. When the adult encounters a fellow-man who is not of the expected mold, he wavers between attitudes of rejection and charity.

Whether he wishes the other well or ill is beside the point; the problem is not at the level of good intentions but at the more obscure level that subtends it. Any human being who makes certain projections impossible because of his condition causes unease in the other—an unease that is denied, and whose effects appear on the Imaginary plane. We have seen proof in the course of history of the meaningless nature of such effects, which have ranged from deportation of alientated persons overseas, to imprisonment under the most inhuman conditions, by way of "medical" attentions of the sort best calculated to strike the imagination. Owing to their very lack of sense, the extreme aspects of such measures point toward the direction we are to follow so that meaning may emerge from the meaninglessness of their coercive nature. The beginning of a more correct approach to lunacy seems to have resulted from the reconsideration of the attitude of the adult confronted with a phenomenon that baffles him, to which he reacts first by resistance.

The situation, subtending as it does an insidious segregation, has something in common with a certain type of racism. What takes place between a racist colonist and a native is not exactly the same as what may take place between a normal adult and a retarded child. To claim that it is, would allow the inference that mental retardation does not really exist. Nevertheless, the question needs to be raised in this roundabout way if we are to grasp the present misunderstanding about retardation. The misunderstanding lies at the very foundation of our ideas about child training and psycho-therapy and deserves to be examined more closely, for it is linked to the possibility of an impasse wherein rehabilitation and psycho-analysis might lose themselves. In my opinion, it is at once neces-sary and urgent to challenge the position of both in relation to the very particular problem of mental retardation, especially at a time when research seems to be losing the impetus given to it by Freud; also, the fact that analysts rarely take part in hospital work leads specialists in maladjusted children to refer to Itard, to Piaget, and to Decroly, rather than to Freud—reducing us at best to pre-analytic methods or their improved versions.

What hampers us today both in pedagogy and psychoanalysis is the dominating influence of developmental theories which take the subject's past history into account only to the extent that favors or hinders "maturation."

A highly questionable parallel is thereby established between physical and mental development. Psychoanalysis has been demon-strating more and more clearly that what matters is not what is given to the subject on the level of needs, but the words, or their absence; it is to words he is referred back by what he is given and by what he feels, thus introducing the field of the Other. Without that, any study of the retarded child is reduced to description in a purely static perspective, discouraging in advance all ideas of prog-ress.

Itard's Mistake

The work of Itard[4] is so misunderstood in our time that it is constantly referred to in the most naive terms, providing a graphic

---

[4] Lucien Malson, *Les Enfants sauvages, mythe et réalité, suivi de Mémoire et rapport sur Victor de l'Aveyron, par Jean Itard* (Paris, Union Générale d'Éditions, 1964). An English version of Itard's book, *The Wild Boy of Aveyron*, was published in 1932 by D. Appleton-Century, New York and London.

illustration of what is still happening today when we face the problem of mental retardation.

The educationalist wants to impose on the retarded child his own concept of the world, and the psychoanalyst is often torn between intellectual curiosity and rejection of the retarded subject who is, so we are told, uninteresting, because of the very poverty of his language. Now, the reason why the experiment with the wild boy of Aveyron is so touching throughout, is precisely because Itard's main concern was to bring him into the world of speech. Yet, Itard's preconceived ideas about the nature of language insured in effect that his pupil's path toward his possibilities would be barred. The mistake is perfectly clear to any psychoanalyst reading this remarkable account, but not to educationalists who are enthralled by the resourcefulness Itard displayed on his mistaken course. It was to Itard's credit that he was willing to embark on something quite new in the way of clinical experiment, but, in his day, it was not possible for him to be sufficiently free of preconceived ideas. His methods can be still detected today as the basis of the most commonly used techniques in remedial work and rehabilitation. Itard's experiment is there to show analysts, physicians, and educationalists that for all the research in this field, they must start first with themselves. What was the trap into which Itard fell at the very outset? Are not his reactions still a determining factor in our own relationship with a retarded child? These are the questions I pose. People hoped in the past that they might receive from the savage the philosophic revelation of man in a pure state of nature, and thought that they could learn everything about it from him. Pinel, on the other hand, regarded the savage as incurably abnormal. Itard's aim was to demonstrate pedagogic resources but in the end he was satisfied with achieving a high degree of training.

Itard had the false notion that Victor lived in a world of pure need (despite all the signs to the contrary, which he honestly recorded), and that he could rehabilitate the boy on that basis. It was not mere chance that he was compared to a severely retarded child.)

Victor was thus first taken up as an object of curiosity and care, to become subsequently an object of remedial measures and it was here that a fundamental misunderstanding occurred.

Victor was not yet able to articulate a demand. This fact seems to have caused Itard anxiety, since it was certainly as a result of the boy's lack of demand that the adult was to assume towards him an attitude of, first, devotion, then rejection, and end up by keeping him out of a sense of duty. The final state of Victor was one of *submission,* and we recognize in it the exact pattern of a certain type of mother–retarded-child relationship, which in effect establishes a sort of subjection of the child to the Other. From the base of having failed to establish a proper human relationship, Itard proceeded to introduce new ideas into rehabilitation methods, the purpose of his theory being—as it had been throughout the past—to compensate for the confusion caused by the adult's helplessness. What we find at the very heart of the problem in Itard's experiment is a failure of communication with the Other.

What do we see on the level of actual observation? An adult confused by a child who does not articulate any demand. From the base of this lack of demand, the adult would like to discover a desire in the child. But it would seem that there is no room for recognizing desire in an adult who is continually referring to need.

To Itard words conveyed the expression of a need. (Victor is imagined saying the word "milk" in order to ask for it.) However, the child used it at will in a game between himself and words. (Milk had an undifferentiated meaning for him; it was a phoneme on the level of which he appeared to maintain himself.)

Itard demonstrates, without realizing it, that the child tended to use language at his pleasure, without making a demand out of it. This was why rehabilitation diminished into mere training.

What Itard had done represented an indisputably enormous advance for his time but, though he fought against existing prejudices in behalf of an admirable faith in human nature, there is a danger that he himself has left a legacy of other prejudices.

We can recognize Itard's ideas in the present situation. Technical advances achieved in the field of rehabilitation under his impetus have nevertheless left open another question: Experience teaches us that rehabilitation proves successful only in cases where beyond the symptom to be remedied, a message is first to be heard; is this not also a subject that deserves closer study?

The first result of our concern for the retarded child was the introduction of an administrative structure to take charge of the mentally defective—in some instances for life. The necessity for administrative machinery must not make us lose sight of its inherent dangers if it is not supplemented by effective clinical research, and all clinical research will prove sterile if it does not begin by self-questioning.

History consists of repetitive behavior. The danger lies in becoming rooted in optimism, in the confident acceptance of administrative procedures, the other side of which is but anxiety and ignorance. The utilization of I.Q. tests often determines the adult's position in relation to the retarded child. Isn't there a place assigned to him from where everything re-enters order? It is from this order in which the child is imprisoned that his adventure begins.

School or Hospital: A Choice
Between Two Evils

Compulsory attendance at school under the present system applies in practice only to children who are regarded as normal. Crowded classes convert the teacher into a mere dispenser of information on the curriculum to those capable of absorbing under such conditions. We have reached the stage of failing to recognize the fundamental problem facing the schoolchild before his apprenticeship with symbols.

The child needs to learn first of all to *see himself* in a way that does not mutilate his being, so as to be able to orient himself with a body he recognizes in space and time, and finally to be ready for *knowledge* which will always be liable to serious distortion if the prelearning required for academic knowledge has not been properly carried through. This applies, of course, in the particular cases where the child has not been able to situate himself correctly on his own in relation to himself and the Other. But all such children do not necessarily require psychoanalysis; between the ages of three and six, they are accessible to influences outside their families in an atmosphere that is not neurogenic. Failure in these early attainments is often the source of reading difficulties, and also the very kernel of a block for the category of slightly retarded children. From preschool age, such children become obsessed by their lack of success; they find themselves at the bottom of the class, or find out what it is to be turned out of a normal school group and wait anxiously to be taken into a special class or a special school for subnormal children.

There are 500,000 intellectually deficient children in France according to current estimates. How many of those children (I am thinking of the slightly retarded and borderline categories) could be salvaged within the framework of normal schooling if we could tackle the problems raised by their difficulties?

The question deserves at least some study. I pose it while at the same time examining the statistical datum which claims that the percentage of mentally retarded varies between 1% and 16%, depending on countries and their political structures.

But, I will be told, you must bear in mind the gap between a highly industrialized and specialized country like England, and one that can still afford to have a large pool of unskilled labor (the Soviet Union has a 1% ratio of mentally retarded).

Such a reply does not satisfy me, because Russia is greatly concerned with the problems of childhood. It has a wide range of well-equipped schools. It is possible for a child to transfer repeatedly between a special school and a normal one, and early vocational training (at the age of nine) is available without excluding academic subjects. Schooling as such does not actually begin before age seven or eight. For four or five years, children learn to observe, to use their bodies; they are introduced to games of physical skill, to dancing, and music. Such a late start in primary education does not prevent them from reaching the level of secondary education at about the same age as do French schoolchildren. The Russian educational system is designed in such a way that children have the impression from their earliest years that they are *working* members of a community. In France, a child who is not gifted academically has to wait until he is fourteen or even sixteen before he is given access to effective vocational training. This means that he is required to passively accept failure and a sort of sterility until that age.

Pierre (twelve years old, with an I.Q. of 70) became both difficult and a bad pupil for that reason. He could barely read or count, "but," said his father, "in the garage, he's the best of the apprentices and the most reliable." After a year's psychoanalysis the boy's I.Q. became normal. Labeled "normal" by a whole battery of intelligence tests, he no longer belonged in the special school for subnormal children which he had been attending.

But where did he belong? Where could he be placed with his low academic level? On his own, the child proposed, "Let me work in the garage and evenings I'll do my school work. I'm sure I'll find it interesting then."

Such a solution is unthinkable under our educational system. It would not be in Russia. In my opinion, this is an unanswered question that deserves further study. Is retardation a constant of nature to be found in all countries, or might there be a sociological factor that favors or hinders the development of a class of handicapped people?

A special school or hospital increasingly tends to be the only choice in France. Does this not mean that a problem that has not yet been studied at the clinical level is subjected to an administrative solution? Is not this solution, like the notions about I.Q.'s, adopted rather hastily to reassure the adult before it has been clearly established what the child gains or loses by it?

Giving Back the Word

The psychoanalytic approach to the problem of mental retardation does not deny that an organic factor plays a role in many cases, but it does not regard this as a basic explanation. Any handicapped person is regarded, above all, as a *speaking subject*. The subject is not a subject of need, still less of behavior, or of knowledge. He is a subject making an appeal by his words, trying to make himself heard (if necessary by a refusal), shaping himself in a certain fashion in his relation to the Other.

He is talking about himself to the Other, and it matters little if he is doing so in a deceiving, touching, colorless, or empty fashion. With a retarded child, as with a psychotic, exact technical conditions are required to bring such discourse out in treatment. This special type of relationship exists in fact between child and mother so that neither can be heard without the other. In serious cases, one may need the support of the other in order to express himself in crude language, or even to remember. At other times, progress achieved by the child can be maintained only if the analyst receives an echo from the parents in the form of a recognition of their own fantasies.

At one point in Mireille's treatment, her mother suffered an attack of depression associated with agoraphobia. It had been the child's task to gratify such attacks in the past. ("What will become of me when I haven't got Mireille any more?"—meaning, when Mireille is cured.) The child, as echo, commented as follows: "When Mummy is sad, she misses having a child. She always wants others to be born so that she feels full, instead of empty and lacking. To be without children makes her unhappy."

In a like response to her mother, Mireille introduced on another occasion the theme of a *doll,* which she needed as a real daughter. "But," she said, "it's easier to talk to a dream dollie. A real dollie can do nothing. A dream dollie can do everything."

The child seemed to be expressing her reply to her mother's

fantasy. She re-enacted with this fetish doll of her own the empti-ness she had to fill in her mother by remaining in her place as the retarded child, and indicated that there was no question of estab-lishing a relation, even an Imaginary one, to the Other. Life is only possible, she seemed to be saying, in a dream relationship, and in any case, isn't a child the remedy against sadness? Where could Mireille possibly have a place as subject in such a relationship?

Nowhere, it seemed, except in the mother, since it was from the time of this depressive episode of the mother that the child lost the use of *I*. And how could she successfully go through the Oedipal experience when the mother herself had not? All these questions form the questions of the treatment itself.

The subject unknowingly reveals a particular form of rela-tionship with the mother (or her substitute) in his words. His "illness" constitutes the very seat of the mother's anxiety, a highly preferential anxiety which cuts across a normal Oedipal develop-ment. The value placed by the mother on a particular type of illness converts it into an object of exchange in a way that perverts, because by refusing a truly triangular situation the child escapes castration at the same time. A certain link with the mother is thus eroticized; this can take place in the first months of the child's life, but it might not occur until after the acquisition of language, or after motor autonomy. A closer study would make it possible to explain the child's preferential choice from among various possible responses.

In cases where an organic factor is in play, the child has to face, in addition to his inborn difficulty, the way his mother makes use of this defect in a fantasy world that will become common to them both.

Leon was four years old and had an irregular EEG. When he was six months old, his parents were told that the child "was im-paired intellectually." He was retarded in his early development, he had insomnia from the age of six months, accepted only liquid food, and did not talk. His tantrums were spectacular. He would sit up, stiffen, scream, and hurl himself backwards. His behavior was quite suicidal. He was unable to express his distress in words, so he tried to destroy himself or some object. The parents were advised to put him in an institution and finally to bring him to me "for a try." The task went beyond a possible organic injury; a meaning in the disturbed mother-child link had to be detected.

Leon was a beautiful child. He refused to walk most of the time, and his mother dragged him or carried him. When he did walk, he was always on the lookout for something shiny, hypnotized by whatever reflected his image—an activity which his mother found hard to take. In all his games, an ecstasy of satisfaction would be succeeded by an overwhelming fit of rage in which he would injure himself. The adult stood by helplessly during these attempts at self-mutilation, because the child's strength increased tenfold, as if he could only find rest after an act of aggression against himself.

The child had a fit of rage of this type in my office during the first interview. I intervened by means of a puppet I called "Gorilla." I said to him, "He's the Gorilla, he isn't Leon." The child stopped screaming at once and began to cry. I hugged him and said: "Dear Leon baby, the son of Daddy and Mummy Rameau." The child calmed down and picked up the puppet. I went on: *"That's* Leon's body, that's the Gorilla, and that [I pointed at another puppet] that's the Gentleman; Leon and the Gentleman aren't the same." The child got up and walked around the room looking for something in which he could find his reflection. "It's the first time a fit of temper has stopped short like that," the mother said emotionally. "I noticed you told him that the Gorilla and the Gentleman weren't him. That must be the important point. As far as I'm concerned, I see and hear nothing but him, and I outscream him, he just drives me to the end of my rope."

In my intervention, I pointed out that *the Other wasn't Leon,* and thereby I introduced into the child's relationship with his mirror-image words that had been lacking. By introducing into language Leon's relation to his own body and to the Other's I broke a certain effect of nonsense in the surrounding discourse in which Leon was always alone, isolated, and hidden. In that place where one is only one, in the most meaningless fashion, Leon was trying to create an Imaginary companion for himself, his double in the mirror. In this narcissistic relationship, the more pleasure he got out of the Other's image, the more an unendurable tension of frustration built up inside him, the only outlet for which was the destruction of the Other or of himself. It was an irruption of anxiety in its most explosive form.

What would it mean if Leon were the Other?—I asked myself. Why is it that as soon as the Other isn't him his attack suddenly stops, resuming normal motility—as soon as his body is situated through my words in relation to the body of an Imaginary companion, to his father's body, and to his mother's? It is as if by means of this fourfold relationship he could free himself from an identification which is cutting him into pieces and mutilating him, because it is situated outside any Symbolic field.

The sessions that followed brought these discoveries: (i) The child recovered his ability to sleep very quickly; the mother said, "Since I have been seeing you, I talk to him; before that, he was retarded, and one didn't speak to him."

(ii) What was to appear next in the mother's words was the extent to which her pregnancy and the death of her father (which occurred during the same period) formed one single event. The child bore the name of the dead father whom the mother was still mourning. "Since his death I've got a lump in my throat; it obsesses me all the time." The father—whom the mother wished to be still living—was seen as present in the son: "He has his hands, his feet."

The question I had asked myself from the outset was, What is the panic that surges up in Leon when he is the Other? Was not the answer, If I am the Other, I am the dead?

What became clear in the mother's case was the impossibility of her having a dialogue with her son; she did not recognize him as a person, as she herself had lost all recognition points by the death of her father. Leon remained for her "a lump in the throat," an alien persecutory body, which is what survived in her of the father she had introjected. Her development as a woman seemed meaningless to her. The child, bearing the imprint of his mother's drama, remained alone with his image which was not mediated by the mother's words, the victim of total panic, for want of the existence of an Other to whom he could refer.

(iii) Leon's insomnia reappeared at a juncture very closely linked to the mother's fantasies of murder and suicide. "I got used to the idea of having a retarded child, it's hard to change." Also she seemed to be introducing something of the order of death in her relationship with the child. "I act as if he didn't exist."

There was no longer any question of "putting the child away" in an institution, according to his doctor, but the mother said to me, tense with anxiety, "If only I could believe he'll get better. I got so used to the idea of getting rid of him."

Both mother and son had a very unusual type of relationship to the partial object. One may wonder whether the child's aggressiveness before the mirror did not correspond to the moment when the subject was able to grasp himself as a unified body. At that moment, his mother conveyed to him very clearly that she wanted nothing to do with the image. Every time the child carried out an experiment leading in the direction of assuming a unified body, the mother let him know that she was unable to assume desire to see him that way, thereby continually sending him back to being only her partial object. The child thus found himself in a situation from which there was no outlet. Any response from his mother referred him back inexorably to the unconscious wish that he die.

This case illustrates what psychoanalysis tries to bring out beyond the reality of an illness, and underlines the importance of the words, or their absence, of those around the child in relation to the medical diagnosis. Owing to the fact that the diagnosis is a severe test for the family, it cannot but take on emotional overtones and indeed occupy a certain place in the parents' fantasy. Only when a painful situation is verbalized, can parents and child attach a meaning to what they are experiencing, and insure that a psychogenic family situation does not arise, as it can only aggravate the child's difficulties in his evolution.

The case also shows that language exists even before the birth of the word. That is to say, it is the exchange between mother and child, beginning at birth, which makes it possible for the baby to structure himself as a person. In the preword language in which they live, there emanates from the mother an ever-renewed gift of life, expressed through words, but also through noises, gestures, rhythms, or simply silence, the silence of peace.

There is an exchange, because the sounds of the child encounter an adult image which sends back the echo of his first cries. It is in this interplay that the desire to use words is born in the child. When this exchange does not take place because of the mother's death fantasies, we will eventually find a being who cannot recognize himself as human. Something on the level of identification can not occur. The child remains mute. He may also develop a form of derangement or intellectual retardation.

The turning point—a chance that he might get better—took place for Leon when he recognized in an animal form that the "bad thing" was not he himself. Giving his badness to an object with which he did not wish to identify enabled him subsequently to begin to speak: "My Manon" (a contraction of "Madame Mannoni"), the child was to say to me one day in a way that overwhelmed me, as we were playing a game of hide-and-seek with our heads, a game in which our voices were silent, but not our hearts.

Acceding to One's Own History

It may happen, particularly in serious cases, that the analyst must talk to the child about the parents' difficulties with regard to their own parents. He thus introduces a dimension that enables the child to situate himself as a link in a chain which is always in a state of becoming. The subject becomes aware that he is inscribed in a line of descent when each person is placed in order in his history. He is then on the path that will give him access to the Symbolic. His recognition points are no longer his real parents, he is in search of a parental ideal as such. He suffers in having to renounce what has been injured in his relation to a parental figure which is contaminating him with anxiety. This mutilated parental figure is received as mutilating for the subject; at this juncture in his analysis, he is facing refusal to accept castration in his own parents.

The analysis of a particular relationship of the child to a progenitor is generally conducted by examining the fantasies he brings up of bodies in bits and pieces. Such fantasies are bulwarks against anxiety. When it proves possible to tackle this form of narcissistic defense in the subject—one which is reactivated when problems of Oedipal identification arise—he can then be led to graft himself in some way onto the image of a sane ancestor, beyond that of the mentally disturbed progenitor. It can be achieved only by the subject's renunciation of a particular period in his childhood, in an idealized relationship with the Other (to whom he is probably the idealized object as well). The child emerges from this narcissistic suffering by situating himself in a line of descent in relation to a sane ancestor, even if he is but fantasy and, in any case, usually dead. Breaking away from impossible identifications, the child can then accede to a mastery of his own past history through a very definite Symbolic dimension. This process offers a chance of successfully treating some children who continue to live in very disturbed homes.

Emmanuel was six years old and unclassifiable. The psychiatrists who had been consulted hesitated between a diagnosis of retardation and one of psychosis. He was severely retarded in his language. The referring hospital wished to avoid institutionalization, which was preferred by the mother.

Emmanuel was described as dangerous; he liked the sight of blood and attacked animals and people. His father was in an asylum. When I asked his mother why she preferred putting her child away to having him psychoanalyzed, I got this answer: "Well, you know, you do things for a man you wouldn't do for a child."

Up to the age of three, Emmanuel had been terrorized by a paranoiac father who would beat him as his mother laughed. The child took the place of an object situated in relation to the parents' sexual relationship; he was the actual center of the couple's gratification. One day, the father tripped him up and said, "Tell me that you'll kill me when you're big, go on, say it." Shortly after, he was taken to the asylum.

Here was a child who had no choice except become his father's murderer or commit suicide, i.e., self-murder. In his behavior, he alternated between destructive conduct and aggression against himself.

Fear of death and castration anxiety were projected on the outside world. Animals, objects, or people thus became persecutory. The child feared that they would penetrate his body. At such times, he tried to keep the other at a distance, as if to safeguard an ideal object within himself. Persecutor and ideal object appeared, however, as two faces of the same figure. Loving and destroying came to mean the same, and the child never knew whether loving (eating) was going to fill him with comfort or discomfort. On the level of interpretation, I always listened to the positive component which formed a part of all attempts at destruction. I introduced words to make it possible for the subject to situate himself in relation to a person who was not suffering from anxiety, one who was capable of resisting the anxiety about annihilation which engulfed the child.

Emmanuel was torn between fear of separation from the beloved object, and the sense of security he seemed to derive from locating a bad object he could control. This was the part played in his treatment by my bringing into the picture something I called "Gorilla"; the child projected on it his uncontrolled and dangerous drives, which represented the failure of all identification.

When he was possessed by Gorilla, Emmanuel suffered anxiety about annihilation. Merely naming it was sometimes sufficient to cut short an attack because, by being named, Gorilla could be situated and controlled in relation to himself.

Whenever the child tried to attack me personally, I verbalized the position of my body and of the objects I liked in the face of attack (saying that I was fond of my body and of the objects around the room, and I would stop them from being destroyed because then they would not be there any more, and I intended to keep them). I intervened by localizing the danger; faced with a given point of reference, the child's anxiety subsided. One might say, he knew that the law of retaliation would not apply. If I refused to be attacked, I would not be the attacker.

On a later occasion, I introduced an interpretation on the level of the subject's wish to return to his mother's tummy, or to eat in order to retain the Mummy he loved. The mother who was beloved was also perceived as dangerous, for the interpretation provoked physical terror. Rolling on the floor, he moaned, "I have tummy ache, I want to go make." Not wishing to expose the child's defenses against frightening words, I put the following question to him: "Do you need to go make, or do you want to make something hurting you inside go away?" With this single question the child was apparently enabled to situate himself in relation to his demand and to my supposed desire. What I was suggesting to him was that I was not the locus of the object of his desire, and that a dialectics of desire was perhaps possible without his having to identify as subject with the partial object.

The child's response to this single remark was to provide material for a considerable number of sessions. He was in fact introducing the point of interdiction related to the demented sadism of his father. It provoked in him a panic that could not be put into words. The child talked to me about people without heads or hearts; it's the only way, he seemed to be saying, that I can manage to live with this insane couple. By losing one's head, one is no longer in danger of understanding; by losing one's heart, one avoids suffering so unendurable that it can find expression only in physical violence.

When I brought into the open the perversion on the father's level, the child asked me for something to drink so pathetically that I could not restrain myself from complying, although I placed "something to drink" in relation to the gift of the mother's presence and the suffering caused by her absence.

From then on, Emmanuel introduced the figure of his mother's sister as a counterbalance to the inadequate mother, and at the same time produced the fantasy of "the tough guy," who had a detachable elastic leg. He had had enough of people laughing at him, and to stop them, in a fit of rage, "he strapped it on." Emmanuel was stressing here his rejection of castration anxiety; his "tough guy," confronted with the Other, demonstrated that he lacked nothing. This theme came up immediately after the revelation of the brutality which the child had been subjected to in reality.

A long period of denial followed; the child could not bear the idea of having mentally disturbed parents, and put himself on the level of their sadism ("It's fun to kill and do naughty things"). To this I invariably answered, "It's sad in your heart to have sick parents." The answer was entirely on the level of the child's defenses, but without laying them bare.

The fact that he had to work through his mourning for a structuring father figure put the child in danger on the level of the castration anxiety, which the mourning seemed to arouse.

The decisive turning point came the day when the child discovered the telephone and created an imaginary telephone for himself. From that moment, he was on a circuit where words were being addressed to an Other, and from the locus of the Other questions could at last stream out. Emmanuel asked himself questions about the origin of the world, generations, and time, and on the meaning of pleasure and pain. He discovered smells, a sense of beauty, ethical values. From then on, he was *educable,* and in analysis he could face symbols; we were in another register, one where words had meaning.

Was he retarded or psychotic? That was the question psychiatrists had asked at the outset.

Emmanuel, first saved from the asylum, now left the special class and returned to normal schooling. He discovered in the analytic situation a witness to his suffering. He received as an echo to his cries words that did not mutilate his being. Access to language occurred as soon as he could invest "naughtiness" in undesirable animal objects; it was the beginning of making a break with impossible identifications. He then had to accept himself as an orphan, and beyond the absence of parents, beyond trials, prove with words his birth and his mastery as subject. And during the years before, it was Emmanuel's bruised body that proved his abandonment and his inhuman loneliness. . . .

When parents and children are confronted with the problem of desire in their relationship to each other from the outset of psychoanalysis, we get from the parents a revaluation of themselves in their own past history; and from the child, asked to speak as subject, we get words which are sometimes so surprisingly articulate that those unaccustomed to this method of analysis wonder whether they spring merely from my imagination.

It may happen that a very handicapped child gives utterance to highly wrought language, even though a moment later he resumes the regressive language by which he is known and loved. Why does he forget in this object relation his state as subject of desire at this point? Why does he respond to what he believes to be his parents' desire by regressing? These are questions to which no reply is to be expected in the near future. I have had occasion to take up with mothers certain bits of their children's speech, and I am always struck by their amazement. "Why does my daughter say 'My father' in talking about her Daddy? Her language is so babyish. It's true," added this particular mother, "that she will always be our baby to us." This remark probably deserves an entire study in itself;

it hints at the importance of the relationship between language and the subject's situation in his interpersonal links. Another mother, obsessed and confused by the idea that her child was retarded, had gone so far as not to talk to him at all during the very important period of his earliest childhood. This may produce superimposed terrors and intractable insomnia in children one to two years old by aggravating their given deficiency, for in order to recognize themselves as human, they always need the adult's words.

Let us listen to Sybille;[5] she was eight years old and had an I.Q. of 50. She appeared as an object to be looked after which relayed her mother's illnesses: "I'm delicate," she told me, "Mummy's very delicate, too. It's not much of a life, always being ill."

"It's not much of a life," the mother told me, "we don't go out any more, everything revolves around the child, we're like a dead family . . . I used to be sickly, they called me a TB germ, but it cleared up with the worry this child gave me. Now that I've put her under your care, I'm ill again like I was before. I feel I'm going to crack up." The exhausted mother waited until her daughter was taken in hand, in order to break down in her turn. In her discourse, the delicate body of one got curiously mixed up with the delicate body of the other. That was my only remark at the third session. At the fourth session, the mother said: "You've opened my eyes, though you haven't given me advice. For the first time, I'm letting Sybille go to the toilet on her own and don't measure her stool any more. Sybille goes out shopping alone, she is trying to break away from us. But, you see, when I let my daughter have her body, I get worn out." When I brought the father into the treatment, I heard this from the child: "You were quite right, Madame Mannoni, to see my father. You should see him a lot. You see, those words which don't mean anything, those nothing words could become Sybille's words." (Sybille was the girl who astonished her mother by using the word "father.")

<hr>

[5] See Maud Mannoni, "Problèmes posés par la psychothérapie des débiles," *Sauvegarde de l'enfance* (January, 1965).

Those words, devoid of sense because they belonged to other people, could indeed become Sybille's own one day. It is the psychoanalyst's job to give them back to the child if he can, and he cannot always. In the psychoanalytic relationship with the retarded or psychotic child, something takes place at a time like that which is of the order of a gift. We have given back to himself the child walled in by terror and petrified in non-communication, so that in his turn he may belong to the world. Though he may be the object of countless attentions, endless solicitude, and the locus of everyone's anxiety, the retarded child sometimes passes unrecognized and misunderstood as subject of desire. Psychoanalytic research makes it clear how much these most underprivileged of human beings have yet to gain by being subjected to a revaluation.

One day in an E.M.P. school[6] in the Paris district, the children were asked to make themselves masks; they were to choose their own designs. Rita expressed the wish in her clumsy language "to have a wall." The educator[7] was not sure that he had understood her correctly and tried to suggest more animate designs. But no, what she wanted was a wall. She *was* in fact the wall, and the adult had to adjust to it. But having it verbally expressed created an uneasiness in the educator along with the awareness that a truth might be concealed in the word. For the psychoanalyst, the anecdote itself is a common one; what is less so, is the effect it had on others. For the child, nothing was changed. The wish had, as it were, escaped her. She would have perhaps found it hard to understand that there was a link between the wish and what she allowed

[6] *Externat Médico-pédagogique* (E.M.P.) is a system of special day schools in France for the education of mentally underprivileged children. The schools have a staff of doctors, remedial specialists, and specially trained teachers and supervisors. (*Translator's note*)

[7] *Educateurs, éducatrices,* are specially trained to superintend the non-academic activities of mentally retarded children, and in some cases act as their teachers. Some are privately employed to look after individual children. This excellent system has been recommended in 1968 by the World Health Organization's Expert Committee on Mental Health for adoption by other countries. (*Translator's note*)

to be seen of herself. But the adult, strangely enough, felt himself accused.

That—the child seemed to be saying—is what you agree that I am. It was the very ambiguity of it that was shocking. It was the child's admission in *words* that pricked the adult's conscience and made him say, "If she says she's a wall, perhaps it isn't so hopeless after all, there must be something behind it." This educator had the merit of being able to accept the pricks of conscience *without resisting* them. Why a bad conscience? Because it was perfectly true that he had had no further hopes for the child.

I am aware of the danger of harm in bringing these questions before members of the public who may feel guilty about them. They will say, "Even if something were feasible, what can we do with the limited resources at our disposal?"—"What's the good of raising hopes, only to say at once that there's a shortage of specialists?"

It is true that courage, which may seem as cruel, is needed to raise a problem publicly when one has only isolated successes to back up one's assertions. But the choice is between this sort of disquiet and a false complacency which is more comfortable but, all in all, more harmful. The most urgent matter is to try to interest the various specialists dealing with maladjusted children in new lines of research. To my mind, there is no question of handing the reins over to the psychoanalysts who, in any case, are basically incapable of meeting the need. But the products of the psychoanalytic attitude in certain cases may be of use to us all in a process of revaluation, and in drawing attention to the possibilities of new discoveries; these are nearer to our grasp than we imagine, provided that hasty answers are not hastily adopted.

BALANCE SHEET OF AN EXPERIMENT IN A SPECIAL SCHOOL[1]

Psychiatrists are in agreement on the need to make hospitals "living, livable, and flexible"[2] before the introduction of individual psychotherapy. When Daumezon embarked on a study of institutional problems, he brought to light an *obstacle:* the existence of "transferences" in the hospital which were diffuse, difficult to situate, and hard to handle. The partisans of institutional psychotherapy then endeavored to work out a theory, making use of the functional elements of individual analysis (transference, countertransference, interpretation). Their aim was to succeed in making the hospital structure itself into a tool for treatment. Their work is marked by the influence of psychoanalysis and is to be distinguished from parallel research carried out (particularly in America and England) by social psychologists. The latter have been accused of not taking into account[3] the unconscious dimension in their

---

[1] Externat Médico-pédagogique, 28, rue d'Estienne-d'Orves, Thiais, Seine. Published in a special number of *Neuropsychiatrie infantile*. The co-operation of staff members made this study possible.

[2] Cf. F. Tosquelles, "Introduction au problème du transfert en psychothérapie institutionnelle," *Revue de psychothérapie institutionnelle*, No. I.

[3] Didier Anzieu, "Étude psychanalytique des groupes réels," *Les Temps modernes*, No. 242 (July, 1966).

studies of real groups (work teams, etc.), which limits their usefulness.

Teams of American psychiatrists and psychoanalysts have attempted to give an account of life in a mental hospital with a wide range of specialists on the staff.[4] They studied the effect on the patient of the way members of the team worked together or against each other, and stressed the part played by the type of relationship between the patient and different members of the staff. "How about patients?" was the humorous question asked by the Chicago hospital team. The patient is seen struggling in the midst of quarrels about theory which are conducted through him, becoming the stake of conflicting psychiatric trends, and, inevitably, the guinea pig for new experiments (specialists in physical medicine, psychoanalysts, and sociologists fighting for the same patient). The hospital is described as a place where diverse influences, opposing interests, and divergent aims collide; the patient is caught in a closely meshed net. The following themes emerge from the studies:

1. The way the hospital functions is closely linked to the needs of all (patients and staff). An institution cannot become a therapeutic place unless it offers the staff not only reasonable living conditions but also chances of promotion and interest in the job. Constant revaluation is needed (both in regard to patients and staff), in order to retain the dynamic dimension necessary for smooth functioning.

2. One of the functions of the hospital is to serve as a "government" for the patients. The details of how the government functions are very important in both practice and theory. The authors regard house rules as therapeutic tools, and illustrate this thesis by a number of clinical examples. The psychiatrist is always closely involved in all administrative decisions (administrative psychiatry is distinguished from psychotherapeutic psychiatry). Whatever

---

[4] Alfred H. Stanton and Morris S. Schwartz, *Mental Hospital* (New York, Basic Books; London, Tavistock, 1954).

the doctrinal positions of the investigators, their inquiries bear on the institutional structure which they endeavor to use as an instrument of liberation for the individual rather than as an instrument of oppression. Various measures are employed. Each team proceeds by trial and error, its experiment being carried out amid difficulties, misunderstandings, and aggressive tensions. Each team seeks to overcome a form of oppression by grasping an institutional reality and by a mastery acquired on the job. It is from this baseline that the team attains the possibility of exchanges on the scientific plane. Work is carried out in an adult environment.

In France, there has been a process of revaluation about institutional structures both for adults and children. Georges Amado's study is relevant in that respect.[5] He has succeeded in putting the problems very pertinently as they appear in the everyday functioning of the school medical services. He provides both an analysis of the situation and a survey of the various unanswered questions. Stress is laid on repercussions at the child's level of any weak spot in the adult.[6]

I. Psychoanalysts in an Institution

The experiment I am going to describe was not particularly original. The institution was small and recently established. It is too early to draw any real lessons from it. It is in my position as psychoanalyst that I am giving a personal account of the experiment, to show what sort of problems confront the psychoanalyst, and not in order to record important results on the institutional level. As far as the relations of psychoanalysts with institutional matters are concerned, two basic ideas are put forth:

[5] Georges Amado, "Douze Ans de pratique médico-pédagogique," in *La Psychiatrie de l'enfant,* Vol. IV (Paris, Presses Universitaires de France, 1961–62).

[6] "As [the director] is with his subordinates, so they will be with the children . . . the children will be with each other, and every child will be with himself. . . . If the children are to have a certain sense of security in an atmosphere of understanding, the members of the staff must feel secure themselves, and have the impression that their essential needs are understood." (*Ibid.*)

1. *Psychoanalysts have no connection with the institution.* They work under the same conditions as in private practice, except that they come to the children instead of the children coming to them. That was our idea at the start. We thought that at the child's level the effect of the difficulties inherent in the institution itself would show up in the child's discourse, and must be heard in their ana-lytic dimension to make treatment possible—a thesis that precluded our intervention in the reality of the child's school life. Often, the child through his symptoms invites the analyst to become involved, and thereby starts up in analysis the game he plays with his parents (a game that serves to mask the Oedipal problems). He sometimes uses his "illness" (and his unhappiness) as his only stake in his rela-tions with other people. The analytic dimension is certainly harder to introduce and maintain in a special school than in private prac-tice. The analyst must be continuously careful to give preference to a certain type of discourse, so that the child succeeds in discerning the symbolic compass of words. The outcome of an analysis is de-cided in the first five sessions and every precaution should be taken from the outset to distinguish it from other kinds of remedial edu-cation. "The drawing for the Gentleman or the Lady" is sometimes requested by four different specialists in the same week.[7] Evidently something in the discourse with the analyst must get recognized beyond the drawing, and interpretations sometimes can be given more quickly in a special school than elsewhere; transference will become established from this juncture (and thereafter, the child will avoid confusing functions and people, by himself).

Being able to hear the parents at the outset of treatment has proved to be of principal importance, especially in cases of psycho-sis. No treatment is undertaken if the parents refuse to come to see the analyst. The psychotic child's speech acquires added signifi-cance when heard with that of the pathogenic parent, as I have shown earlier. The interaction between their words very quickly

---

[7] We should rethink the various forms of remedial education, as the need for educators who are generalists is making itself felt. The division into multiple specialties is of no advantage to the child.

gives the analysis its precise dimension. The essentials of the parents' Oedipal problem emerge in the first ten sessions. (The child's Oedipal situation becomes clearer when it is seen in the light of the parents'.)

The analytic dimension can be preserved only by a certain strictness, which is not a question of *attitudes* (kindly, severe, aloof, friendly), but one of selecting what is to be regarded as preferential in the discourse. Thus, a case is to be made for psychoanalytic consultations in the environment of a special school; all that is required is to define the context within which one is to function.

In regard to the analyst's relations to the establishment, it would be naive to suppose that all he has to do is act discreetly so as not to alarm the adults concerned. It is no good his trying to break down the barriers, his presence will make itself felt. His own feelings of guilt about the damage he may cause only increase the persecutory anxiety of the group. He is an intruder, to a far greater extent than any other colleague. It is not his presence in reality that is oppressive. The burden lies in what the analytic myth represents in the adults' unconscious. It is the adults who stick the label of "analyst" on him, and it would be a mistake to believe that he can lose it by making people "forget" him—I almost wrote "forgive" him—with friendly gestures. The psychoanalyst is *for the Other,* the one who is deemed to know. It might even be said that he owes the essential part of his influence to the fact that there is always a believer in analysis; this suffices to force him to play the game, to support the aggressive and persecutory projections of his co-workers, whom he *puts in danger* in exactly the same way as psychoanalysis puts those who engage in it in danger. An emerging truth is encountered here, despite a widespread tendency to keep it veiled. In essence, this feared truth is the confrontation of the unconscious with the Oedipal myth.[8] I can now formulate the second proposition without contradicting the first.

---

[8] It is not uncommon in private discussions with the analyst for an educator spontaneously to associate the difficulties a child raises in him with his own Oedipal problem, approached through the problem of death.

If the analyst does not concern himself with the institution, the institution will concern itself with the analyst. To show just what the problem is, I will try to describe how things came to be more or less worked out through adjustments in a small institution. I will attempt to make clear the questions the analyst finds himself asking.

The special school is authorized to accept mildly and moderately retarded children with serious behavior problems. Out of approximately forty children between the ages of six and fourteen, about a quarter are psychotics. There are two preschool classes and three school classes, extending in theory from first grade through eighth grade. The standard, however, is very low, barely going beyond the middle grades.

Before the school was officially established, there was in Paris a nucleus of educators teaching handicapped children under adverse material conditions. There was no proper structure of medical administration. The dedicated and efficient teachers did their best for the children entrusted to their care, but working conditions were difficult and the lack of accommodations restricting. The official establishment of the school was awaited with a mixture of hope and fear. The prospect of administrative supervision and medical control appeared fettering. Nevertheless, when the institution was launched, the teaching staff was solidly behind it. The material difficulties they had to put up with temporarily, as the building was not yet equipped to fully accommodate the children, strengthened their solidarity. Children *and* adults had to face the same inconveniences, and this is an important point to which I shall return later. Cramped quarters, the noise of builders, imperfect heating, all formed part of "hostile nature," and adults and children entered into battle to overcome the obstacles. The special school was born imperceptibly; during the early days, the team of educators carried out the job of moving into a building full of workmen.

The problem of really becoming organized did not arise until the second year of the school's existence. From the material viewpoint, everything was at last ready to deal efficiently with defective children. The educators were no longer on their own as the traditional specialists gradually arrived, ranging from school secretary to physician-in-chief. Administrative measures made themselves felt in the form of various restrictions. A group could no longer "become official" without submitting reports on a variety of matters. The introduction of a physician-in-chief altered the purely educational nature of the place; it represented a challenge to accepted customs. The birth of a special school, like the birth of a child, never turns out quite as you expect it. There is always a gulf between what *reality* has to offer and what is invested on the fantasy plane. The wider the gulf, the greater the feeling of a lack that is impossible to fill; the situation will then be lived in a persecutory mode (the feeling of having been swindled in carrying out a project). During this stage of the launching, the adults experienced a certain amount of confusion. For the first time, they were really alone with their problems. The tension caused by a hostile outside world had dissolved, and in its place came a vague, ill-defined tension within the staff.

No one, to begin with, was really conscious of uneasiness, but the signs heralding it were discernible nevertheless. The adults feared contacts with the outside world; any incursion by outsiders was resented as an extra strain. Little by little, communication within the group of educators faded out, and there were moments of blockage that were experienced by some in a particularly acute way. This eventually affected communication between some of the adults and the children. It was at this point in the crisis that the psychoanalytic team came on the scene. They came in fear of disturbing an adult environment drawn within itself. They settled themselves into a watertight compartment beside the group already in another watertight compartment. It was like an autonomy moving in on another autonomy. The uneasiness became marked on the part of both educators and analysts. The latter, while representing advanced ideas in the theoretical realm, failed utterly in integrating into the life of the school. As the effects of the uneasiness were felt at the children's level, we started to do some soul-searching. Analysis is not possible in an oppressive atmosphere; what were we doing that contributed to such an atmosphere? We had a share in it. The group had made itself its own oppressor and thus cut itself off from the children. In an adult environment, there is always a "persecutor" who is regarded as being the major cause of strain. Everyone feels himself "put upon" or "tricked" by the other. The third element in the relationship with the Other abruptly disappeared to be replaced by a dual type of situation that introduced a pathogenic factor. The devastating effects it produced were felt at all levels.

II. Entering into a Situation

The staff members were in the grip of anxiety. At the beginning unity was secured on the basis of an ideal. The school's evolution involved new goals (the quest of another ideal), which aroused resistance among some people, causing a form of encapsulation. Sometimes, the paralysis of one member in a team is sufficient to cause a communication block. (Usually the ego-ideal has been wounded, leading to a stream of complaints and a sort of moral abdication.) The entry of psychoanalysis can be compared to focusing a searchlight on the disorder, but it is to no purpose until the analyst joins in the transference with his own set of problems. The analyst-observer is resented as a voyeur, a spy, either associated with someone trying to steal the "good object," or else with the "bad object" to be discarded. The position of observer is a destructive one, because it does not permit the verbalization of unconscious fantasies. The analyst is unknowingly trapped in the net of an Imaginary fascination which he cannot control, as he cannot anticipate the depressive and persecutory stances such a situation will engender. The analyst who is not integrated with the adults in an organization can only observe a group's pathology; he is incapable of anticipating its effects. The place we had assigned him *outside* the group, even if it had meaning at the children's level, had none at all at the adults' level. It was as analysts that we had to embark on some type of relationship with everyone individually, so as to free them from their fantasies and imaginary snares. This entailed a self-searching on the part of the analyst with regard to his own countertransference on the institution.

It was understood by the physician-in-chief that individual psychoanalysis in an institution had no meaning unless it was integrated with the institution as a whole. Some structure was needed, which had to be built up from scratch. Struggles for prestige and aggressive relationships could not continue any longer without the danger of making our work sterile, and the effects of that could not fail to have repercussions at the children's level. The analysts offered the image of a dynamic team centered on clinical work and research, their productive activity cutting across that of the educators who were isolated in their difficulties. A team concept seemed to us tenable within the general context of the school only if the analyst responsible for his own group (myself, in this instance) became part of the institutional organization. The purpose of this was not only to re-establish a communication circuit but also to insure that there would be a policy on matters of common interest (questions of theory, scientific research), and on a practical level (reconsidering accepted practices).

What type of mediation could we introduce?

The problem was to be examined from the starting point of this question. It was necessary to reintroduce a ternary dimension (a verbal one), which had disappeared in the type of relations instituted among the adults, as well as between adults and children.[9] For that purpose, it seemed useful to focus the interest in discussions among educators on research projects which originated in *obstacles* they had reported. The impasse in teaching activities, school

[9] This third dimension consisted in referring adults and children back to more important considerations and interests which would dictate the style of their mutual relations.

organization, and material problems had caused panic among the adults and referred them to problems situated elsewhere than where the apparent difficulty was (the link with a form of persecutory anxiety is obvious). If the fantasy elements underlying the obstacle are not flushed out, there is the risk of stereotyped reaction-formations which close the door on any possibility of inquiry, that is, on true research. (The wish to "reorient" some children may be based on a record of educational failure which is worth examining. Scientific mastery is possible only after analysis of the failures and successes. Any analysis of this sort implies a *situation* involving teacher *and* pupil, and should be examined as such.) The analyst's intervention may remain on an apparently superficial level; it is sufficient in the course of discussion to keep the options open in cases where a final and categorical answer was returned previously. He thus leaves everyone with the chance that the play of substitute signifiers may occur (the time needed to understand is not the same for everyone). Such a demand for reorientation touches on the adult's anxiety in the face of the unbearable anxiety emanating from the child. If one can contrive to formulate it in the form of the question, "To whom shall we give Fanny?" (meaning, How can we get rid of her and of our own anxiety?), a register is reached in which it is already no longer necessary to "give" the child, because what is implied in the demand has already been recognized.

Progress meetings with the analyst were intended to secure the requisite conditions under which research could be carried out. A phenomenological procedure is possible only if the educator does not feel himself at fault for having failed. It is his feeling of guilt that leads him to suggest concrete measures where investigations should be made.

Progress meetings without the analyst (with the attendance of the physician-in-chief) made it possible to draw up a plan for theoretical study based on evidence supplied by the educators. (The latter also met informally to discuss it among themselves.) The results of this work were kept "secret" from the analyst for a while. Time was needed before the educators were willing to situate their evidence in the locus of interchange. So long as the work was not made available to the entire community, it was devoid of any real scientific value, and the conception of a team assumed its full meaning only when the pedagogic impact could be studied in the light of the other disciplines. (This form of resistance was in effect the expression of resistance to psychoanalysis only, to which the analysts themselves had contributed by not embarking on a dialogue from the outset.) Work and research subsequently became mediators in interpersonal links.

However, individuals made an *oppressive* use of them during the first phase, because they were not consciously used in the service of liberating each of us. Educational problems were tackled as a function of the personal position of the adults in relation to their work. The team's inclination in relation to the children was probably to individual teaching, which raised specific difficulties in cases of psychosis and serious behavior problems.[10] The class conceived as an organized group forms a framework within which it is possible to entrust a team of children with the task of working out a class project. This permits the structuring of a situation where the relation is to work, and no longer to people. Teacher and pupil escape thereby from the depressive and persecutory anxiety engendered by all dual situations. This concept of teaching, which has been found to work elsewhere,[11] is now under study in this special school. Resistance to its application is due in part to difficulties of a technical nature (too little space and equipment, and too few educators), in part to difficulties of a psychological order, namely, that a community system of education makes the educator question the place he occupies in a hierarchy founded on authority. The participation of

[10] Some children who are particularly resistant to academic schooling seem open to early vocational training; unfortunately, it can be given only on a part-time basis.

[11] In a series of special classes in the Paris region.

pupils in organizing a class project puts the teacher in the place of a group leader rather than that of undisputed authority. The experiment was tried out from time to time with some educators, and it demonstrated that they occupy a key position in the situation. In order to adjust his way of speaking to the situation in which he is involved, the educator himself must not be driven by his own unconscious processes. If he loses control of them, he may suffer a disturbance which is liable to have effects at the group level. The intervention of an analyst may then help the educator to put into perspective the situation in which he is imprisoned. The risk of disturbance is decreased if the analyst is not blindly caught up in the play of his own countertransference. The child can have the benefit of a whole series of reactions, if the educator retains sufficient mastery of the situation.

The therapeutic effects of this pedagogic conception are worth studying through the cases of success and failure. In undertaking class projects, many problems had to be reconsidered (from educational obstacles, to the delicate problem of professional orientation, and even including questions of physical organization in the building). Everyone, at various junctures, was impelled to revise his positions, and there was a move towards the overthrow of the ego-ideal (in correlation with a new status involving everyone when the school became an officially organized place); but this did not come to pass without a serious crisis, and some people, in fear of losing their own identity, tended to invite the very exclusion they dreaded, which was in line with their anxiety about being abandoned. In an evolutionary situation, a group is liable to show itself intolerant of anyone unconsciously putting a brake on the chances of progress. Team life has moments of intense anxiety, associated with individual projections of fantasy. A disturbed personality can accentuate the collective anxiety by bringing home his own terror to each member; this can lead to situations where the group seeks to expel one of its members. The physician-in-chief played a key role here in damping emotions by the right words (touching on persecutory anxiety). The team, paralyzed by the imaginary terrors they had created out of nothing, were then able to overcome them. Conflict situations became easier to control, as bases for work and research were more solidly established. The preservation of a Symbolic dimension prevented acting-out.

III. The Clinical Problem

This could be considered more rationally from the base of the first revaluation. What could we do to insure that the atmosphere of the special school offered children the chance of improving? If children and staff contributed to the creation of misunderstandings, they ought to be able to contribute to their solution also.

There seemed to be two forms of intervention: (i) dealing directly with the disturbed children (this was the analysts' job); (ii) dealing with what was happening among the staff (this was the job we were to share with the physician-in-chief).

Collaboration with the educators proved valuable in the case of psychotic children. They sometimes carried to the classroom the play of analytic transference, trying to express in reality what they could not make happen in the Symbolic register. (Melanie Klein calls this type of transference "psychotic transference.") Discourse begun in treatment was then replayed in the institution as a whole. We witnessed a series of lateral transferences which were interesting to make deliberate use of. The classroom atmosphere in a special school is a locus of investments and identifications (for children among themselves and for children with adults).

Psychotics have preferred places, for example, the kitchen, and the part played by the cook sometimes proves to be a very important one. (It should also be possible for her to be heard by the analyst, inasmuch as she accepts the strain of anxiety by putting up with the presence of disturbed children.)

It is important to safeguard in some corner of the establishment a chance of expression in a context that is not abnormal. Words blocked in the classroom can be taken up again elsewhere, but this has no structuring effect unless it can take place within a framework where the institution provides for participation in communal activities, when the child is absent from classroom activities. (Some children become easier to return to the classroom after they have spent some time in the kitchen.) The adult's threshold of endurance must be respected, however. It can only be regretted that there are no arrangements for activities that would make it easier to return to the classroom children who are resistant to schooling. Being a pupil has no meaning as part of the learning process, unless it makes possible the introduction of the third dimension, so basically lacking in the psychotic.

In conducting treatment, it is not necessary for the analyst to be told about the continuation in the classroom of discourse begun in a session. But from the institution's point of view, it is not unhelpful if the analyst knows about the blocks of some children or the acting-out of others. Such reactions are often directly associated with an emotional situation in the institution, which the child perceives. If the educator in charge of the child is himself rejected by the group, the child will directly suffer the effects of this. No sooner had a teacher said to me, "I can't communicate with anyone any more," than a child told me in reference to him, "I can't talk to my teacher any more, it's all over." I went into the problem with the teacher and brought to light a persecutory element in him, related to exclusion mechanisms that led him to establish false relationships with adults and children. Neurotically exercised authority has perverting effects, owing to the sadomasochistic relationships it sets up. When the functions of authority are perverted, there is no longer a reference to the Law as the guardian of order; the relations of subjects to each other are reduced to the dimension of a dual situation, the pernicious consequences of which we have already studied.

The administrative organization of an institution must be constantly rethought in relation to its order and disorder. It is better if the rules themselves do not remain static but change in accordance with the needs of a progressing group. The experiment made us subscribe to a truth well known by those who work in a hospital atmosphere, namely, that an institution has viable existence only if patients and staff find in it the means of making progress. When communication is no longer blocked at the adult level, then, and then only, can the children have a chance of expression. To prevent an institution from closing in on itself, each of its members must be guaranteed the chance of projecting to the future. The participation of everyone in scientific work is in itself therapeutic; following through a piece of research properly presupposes in effect the setting aside of personal conflicts, and the continuity of discourse is guaranteed.

IV. The Purpose of the Special School

The school treats children in difficulties, but also functions as a *research and training center for young analysts*. There are insufficient funds to pay specialist staff properly, and the location of the school in a suburb which is difficult to reach adds to the problem. However, by offering young people training, not a job, by giving them an opportunity to do clinical work under supervision, and by making them part of a research team, recruits of a high caliber can be secured. The formula of providing free training cannot, however, remain the solution for the future; it is a temporary expedient.

Candidates must be serious about the work. It happens sometimes that young inexperienced people are as effective as old hands (provided, of course, that they are being analyzed). The aggressive projections of certain psychotics have the effect of making them revaluate their own positions with regard to the signifier (death, Name of the Father, etc.). The fact that they have been marked by the child's anxiety becomes a valuable tool in the treatment, as the child is brought to life from the base of the analyst's desire. What may appear to be ill-timed or clumsy interventions by a trainee can be useful if the supervisor helps him situate in his own personal problems the particular words on which he has embarked with the child. Thereafter, he will be able to find for himself the right words in a situation that was calculated to catch him unawares at the start.

Our special school thus pursues parallel research in education and psychoanalysis. We endeavor to maintain general agreement as to the direction of the work. It is certainly not an easy undertaking, and disputes about theory easily arouse strong feelings. It is essential, as we have seen, that concern for the work be introduced in interpersonal relations as a third point of reference. The adults' discourse is thereby constituted with reference to a common research. It would be naive to suppose, however, that all problems are solved because considerations of a didactic nature have been introduced into the group. Let us rather say that they provide a less deadly and more useful battleground than dueling in a situation of mirror-aggressiveness. The adults are given the opportunity to talk to the analyst about the effect which the tensions of institutional surroundings have on them, and conflicts become less acute. An analytic outlet does not remove the tensions and difficulties of group life, but it makes it possible to take the drama out of some misunderstandings caused by a fantasy element on a persecutory theme. All work teams have their quota of difficulties and inevitable clashes, which are in effect prerequisites of progress, but it is essential that their discourse not become blocked. This is why a ternary mediation proves indispensable.

To sum up, we entered a situation as analysts, and we were marked by the effects of tension in institutional surroundings. The effects can be productively studied at two levels: (i) bringing to light each adult's countertransference on the institution; (ii) understanding the adult's reactions of identification or counteridentification with the "illness" of a certain type of child.

The study has an experimental value in that our choices and options are functions of our training and our way of thinking, but also of our defenses. Published studies[12] on institutional problems throw light on the difficulties of living in a shut-in atmosphere.

[12] Cf. various issues of the *Revue de psychothérapie institutionnelle.*

The gulf between the world of the "sick" and the world of the healthy[13] is one which we have introduced as protection against our own fear. Experience shows us that a therapeutic approach is possible only if we become part of the "sick" man's world. But then we run the risk of being savagely assaulted in our being by the projections of psychopathic subjects. Some protection is therefore necessary, but it does not lie in the judicious use of the couch, nor in keeping up a highly organized hierarchical structure. It lies in the technical means at our disposal to maintain discourse at a controllable level (by providing it with a third dimension). The analyst learns such control the hard way when he begins to be responsible for directing treatment. He also learns the hard way when he embarks on the adventure of community living. He cannot maintain himself in the place of a mere observer, he must share in the common tension; but sharing it as analyst presupposes his control over discourse which has a tendency to become debased unless it is kept in a Symbolic dimension that guarantees the order of language. The words that the child is trying to speak will be situated in this order (or chaos). What he hears in the adult world may cause the child to work out a deranged type of discourse; the atmosphere of the hospital or school may also deepen in certain types of children the imprint left by a form of family derangement.[14] This spells out the importance to be attached to the institutional structure before undertaking individual treatments there.

[13] Thomas Szasz, *The Myth of Mental Illness* (New York, Hoeber-Harper, 1961; London, Secker & Warburg, 1962).

[14] Laing and Esterson, *Sanity, Madness, and the Family.*

THE DIFFICULTIES OF COLLABORATION BETWEEN PSYCHOANALYSTS AND EDUCATORS IN INSTITUTIONS[1]

Difficulties arise when the difference between the *educational* position and the *analytic* position has not been clearly defined at the outset. In the first case, a work of adjustment is being organized around the *reality* of the retarded or psychotic child; in the second, our inquiry starts from the base of our own *representation* of the child. In our relation to the child, we know that the subject is generally in a place *other* than where he appears to us. The art of analysis lies precisely in being able to summon him from that other place where he has fled both from us and from himself.

If one sticks to this basic difference, one is reduced to a traditional pedagogic conception that keeps the two disciplines distinct in watertight compartments. But one may wonder whether there is not in fact an interaction between psychoanalysis and education; if that be the case, there are probably grounds for second thoughts on educational methods in the light of psychoanalytic discoveries.

"The psychology we are taught," a teacher admitted, "seems

[1] Extract from an article published jointly with M. Safouan in a special issue of *Recherches* (September, 1967), entitled "Enfance aliénée" (preparatory work for an international symposium on psychoses, Paris, October, 1967). We owe our experience of educators to the educators themselves: Mmes. Dubois, Marteau, Raynaud, and Hamele; Messrs. Billiet and Brochard.

completely wrong to us from the moment we discover in a book what analysts are saying. As soon as everything we had been taught proves to have been wrong, we can't go on teaching." [2]

We must, of course, distinguish between the situation where the educator may feel uneasy with the idea of psychoanalysis as he conceives it or as he got it out of a book, and one where gaining access to his own unconscious may have produced certain effects on him. It is from the base of the effects of confronting what has been repressed that the specialist revaluates his work in his own field. He is impelled to rethink what has been handed down to him in a particular cultural tradition, and to contrast received instruction with a basic revaluation of himself in his job. "Am I there to transmit knowledge, and what is one transmitting when one thinks one is teaching?" Would it be advisable to separate the idea of *education* from that of teaching?

In primitive societies, language and duty towards one's parents were not the concern of education.[3] The subject of teaching was myths, and the dominant force in a certain form of social tradition was the mystification of children. The *mystifying factor* in the adult-child relationship still exists unrecognized in our day, and it supports a great many of the prejudices about education. It is from this starting point that a new type of educational activity might be devised in which, for example, room might once again be found for teaching myths.

The educator is in a different position from the analyst, because he does not question his relation to *desire*. The analyst is essentially concerned with everything that touches on his own relation to truth. Nevertheless, an educator affected by analysis would more easily have access to the right words, which cannot be taught, but which surge out of the personal experience of an adult aware of the child within himself.

---

[2] J. Danos, October 6, 1966, at a working meeting on methods of teaching psychotics.

[3] O. Mannoni, at a working meeting on methods of teaching psychotics, October, 1966.

If the teacher's position is different from that of the analyst, the problem of teachers and psychoanalysts co-existing in an institution arises at quite another level.

Even the term "collaboration" evokes the idea of watertight disciplines, gathering in plenary session on the subject of "the child." In this perspective, the analyst appears as yet another specialist, coming to swell the ranks of speech therapists, occupational therapists, and a variety of remedial specialists. Shut up in his own special field, he remains deaf to what is going on in the institution; he thinks he can work there as he can in his office, without realizing that there, more than anywhere else, he is part of the machinery in a system which he will find himself forced to question. It is a fact that the analytic dimension is harder to preserve in sessions in an institution than outside. The child, caught between a ball game, a session with the lady who does speech therapy, another with the lady who does psychology, and the routine interview with the physician, is not always sure what he ought to be talking about with the analyst—neither what, nor to whom. Therefore, individual psychoanalysis in an institution is not possible, unless there is rethinking about the basic structure of the establishment. This point of view has been stated by many, and developed at length by not a few. Our concern is more modest, in that we do not want so much to make the institution therapeutic in itself as to insure that the work done in treatment is not undone in the institution, because its structure, or lack of it, is closely akin to family structures that produce psychosis. We have given an account earlier of putting an analytic spotlight on an institution; what we are attempting to define now is the *situation* of the teacher, as a certain analytic approach has revealed it. Our field of study is very limited; we propose to offer only specialized education for children resistant to normal schooling. The traditional position is based on criteria of adjustment, and adjustment being postulated as an end in itself constitutes by that fact the major obstacle we have to contend with. Faced with the difficulties of a psychotic child, the teacher can see for himself the bankruptcy of principles that underlie his theories. He then begins to revaluate these principles along with the instruction that has been given him. In search of other guidelines, he turns to psychoanalysis.

It was belief in the physiological origin of psychiatric disorders that provided education with its medical bases. In this perspective, educational techniques aim essentially at carrying out special compensatory training, which will result in relative adjustment. It is, of course, the educator who *desires* this relative degree of adjustment, and decides what it shall be. He believes that he is taking into account the needs and interests of the child, without suspecting that these needs and interests are, above all, his own as an adult. He assumes that the child has his own representation of the world of childhood; very often, he is unaware of what in himself may be challenged when he encounters a psychotic. The outcome may be his failure to recognize the child as the subject of words or desires. The analyst's contribution may be to impel the educator to rethink his whole mode of being with the psychotic. He can give the "right" response to the child only from the base of how he, the adult, feels implicated in some way in the symptom. Ordinary educational methods do not work with the psychotic. Learning refers him back to a danger—that of being trapped as an unintegrated body in the adult's dialectics. Alienated as subject, the psychotic presents himself successively as a mouth to be fed, an anus to be filled. He encourages a purely mothering relationship and becomes petrified in a sort of body-to-body association. The problem then confronting the adult is how to make the child enter the order of desire. How can he be got to overcome the stage of a stereotyped, constantly repeated demand?

It is when the adult is able to give up making direct demands, thereby bringing the child's body into play, that a *non-dual* situation is established and gives *desire* a chance to be born between educator and child. It is also necessary, in order that the situation acquire structure, for desire to be symbolized; that is to say, something in relation to words is to be organized, thus establishing in the child the meaningful word of the unconscious. In the customary relationship between educator and psychotic child, the latter is told to "do this" or "do that," without being able to give a meaning to the adult's message. It is precisely this imaginary derangement that must be overcome. (It is, of course, the psychoanalyst's job in the management of treatment, but he can receive great assistance from the surroundings, i.e., the *words* in which the child is caught up.)

When the institution is entirely centered on the child, he may feel himself trapped in its demands. In fact, the psychotic, more than any other child, needs the educator to be interested in something other than him. To do this, the whole art is to succeed in directing the child's desire towards something other than the adult himself.[4] Educators point out, in illustration of this recoil into himself, the ease with which the psychotic child (if he is not completely shut in autism) imitates what a classmate is doing, any classmate. He goes from one imitation to the other, from one mask to the next. He never really enters into a structuring form of identification. To have a chance of such identification, the child must be able to distinguish himself from the other. The psychotic child does not make this distinction. He remains highly dependent on desires stemming from maternal omnipotence. When he speaks to us, either he situates us in himself or he voices words which are not his. This is not, as one might be tempted to think, a problem of *communication,* but of the child's very relation to language. This is where we must study the meaning of the adult message which is, or is not, "passed on." The adult-child misunderstanding is, in the case of psychosis, always fundamental, since the adult as the Other is totally ruled out by the child. We can see the effects on educators of being cancelled out in this way. The effects are translated into words. From the base of words, the child in his turn conducts the game. "I'm lost,"

---

[4] This is the interest of contributions to educational techniques, such as that of Freinet, studied and applied in particular by F. Oury and Aïda Vasquez (thesis on "La Pédagogie institutionnelle," June, 1966). See also their *Vers une pédagogie institutionnelle* (Paris, F. Maspero, 1967).

Carole asserted just when the educator told us, "We'll never get anywhere." We were faced here with a crisis for child *and* adult. By understanding what was in play in this situation, the educator was able not only to find the right words but also not to repeat parental behavior with the child. (In this case, not to refer her any more to her mother's remark, "You're pushing me to the end of my rope," which only increased the child's violence in the grip of anxiety roused by her murderous fantasies.)

In experiencing in an institution the adventure of "learning" for handicapped children, we begin to rethink the entire problem of learning in school, in relation to the nature of the obstacles encountered. The overwhelming part played by the interrelation of the child's difficulties with their effect on the adult's unconscious stresses the importance of psychological factors in all educational methods. We found that the role of psychoanalysis in an institution was not only treating children (where it might be reserved for the serious cases), but, above all, in analytic listening to the educators. It ought to be possible to devote some time to the adults who are the support of the child's anxiety. Besides, it reduces the risks of attacks of depression and depersonalization among educators who are all too often exposed in their being (without the protection conferred by a personal analysis) to the aggressiveness or apathy of a certain type of child. The analyst can give the educator the insight that permits him to adjust what he says to a situation, the meaning of which escapes him insofar as he is implicated in a way he does not appreciate.

In this perspective, we saw how education was transformed as soon as it left the traditional atmosphere. The transformation was accomplished as soon as education took its place in a collective discourse, with the analyst present. But this presupposes that the necessary institutional structure has already been built up. If this has not been done with the complete agreement of the administration, the experiment might easily fail. In the discourse that will go on at the institution, something will come into play at the level of reshaping a being. The educator, in his difficult and unrewarding work, understands the benefit he derives from such a type of relationship. Through it, he will attain real mastery in his work.

But this is not sufficient. The institution does not consist solely of analysts and educators, and one soon discovers that the Oedipal drama is being played out in it. The institution must stage-manage it. When the institution fails, it means that the administrative structure has failed (by being inadequate) to allow technical control of emotional situations brought on by a sort of liberation of adults or children in the institution. If the administrative structure is reformed in such a way that everyone becomes personally involved, then it is not possible to have a phony institutionalization. Full access by the teaching staff to a form of personal mastery forces the school administration to join in the game as well (i.e., to rethink their functions on the basis of an institution which, by choice, remains unossified). The traditional hierarchies, as Jean Oury has demonstrated on several occasions,[5] maintain a form of dependence that gives preference to a very special type of relation in which everything centers around the demand on the other and of the other. This structure keeps up a masochistic type of relationship and breeds acting-out, which always affects the children. When a proper analytic standpoint is introduced into an establishment, sooner or later some staff members ask for a personal analysis. It is impossible in such a situation for an administration to remain isolated, outside the transformation affecting all the adults in the school. The result of such isolation would be a cell of resistance in the institution itself, which would create a feeling of insecurity among the staff and have unfortunate repercussions on the progress of psychotherapy. If the "freed" words of children and educators cannot be taken up elsewhere at the same level of interchange, they produce a blockage which gives rise to acting-out in the adult sphere.

This concern with the proper setup of an institution is, of course, somewhat utopian. As analysts, we know that the subject is always in some place other than where he appears in his responsibility and

[5] Jean Oury, at a working meeting on institutional problems, December 1, 1966.

his adjustment. He can be truly summoned only in individual treatment. Even the most smoothly running institutional machinery always has something contrived about it, always endeavors to conceal that it has an impossible dimension within itself. It is nonetheless true that once the analytic standpoint has been introduced into an institution, it will no longer be possible for the educators to work under other conditions. The benefit they derive from it may be compared with the effects of a personal analysis. We do not wish to imply that an institutional reorganization ought to dispense personal analysis; still, one cannot fail to be favorably affected as the authentic word emerges through all sorts of blocks in this type of collective discourse.

The educator understands for himself that he should situate the psychotic in a life style with a varied range of investment. This is where teaching stops.[6] The aim with the psychotic child is not to train him but to integrate him into a reality provided by institution life (cleaning, cooking, washing up, running errands, shopping), and children mixing with each other on the basis of tasks undertaken in common. The educator's demand will no longer be directed at the child, but towards the machinery of everyday work in which he will find himself caught up. A certain flexibility of behavior will encourage the adult to follow up some children in what they are trying to do in directions other than where the adult's demand pins them down. The teacher's discoveries with this type of child (arising from attentions before the possibility of formal schooling exists) are always situated in the domain of what the child does not succeed in doing.[7] What we should pay heed to is what the child brings when the adult is not expecting it.

The more we progress in our work at the institution, the more convinced we remain that the effectiveness of analysts in an establishment lies neither on the level of merely conducting individual

[6] Ginette Michaud, at a meeting in December, 1966, on institutional problems.
[7] O. Mannoni, "Itard et son sauvage," *Les Temps modernes,* No. 233 (October, 1965).

treatment nor on the level of a so-called dialogue with the educators. An analytic standpoint must be introduced at the level of the institution, and the educator will be able to make his own discoveries there. Psychoanalyst and teacher should not take up positions like two workmen working around the same object, but as custodians insuring the proper functioning of the institution. It is in this way that the educator can teach and the psychoanalyst can think about his individual cases. In an institution, psychoanalysis and education should not co-exist as different disciplines, side by side with all other therapies, parceling the child out to a large number of specialties. Psychoanalysis has meaning only if it can be conducted from a position where the analytic spotlight makes it possible to change the language of education. Freud faced the same question; he saw that the task of the analyst and the educator are by nature different, and said so, but he could not suggest any solution other than offering the educator the benefit of personal analysis. This is obviously a solution, but one that is cumbersome to the point of being impracticable. In an institution, it would soon become clear that the same procedure would have to be applied to all concerned, without taking into account the additional difficulty that analysis is valid only if it has been asked for. In any case, it is clear from Freud's position that there is absolutely no question of turning the educator into an analyst. To start with, their work is basically different. Freud merely wanted the educator to have been analyzed. Although we do not think it necessary to insist on that, we do insist on the beneficial side effects produced by the analytic position in an institution.

These questions have not been examined in sufficient detail. It is not a matter of collective psychotherapy or of group analysis, but of something more subtle that the analyst comes to feel when he works in an institution; he is obliged to take it into account, for he always meets it first of all in the unpleasant shape of obstacles, resistance, or aggressive demands.

BIBLIOGRAPHY

Abraham, Karl, *Dreams and Myths: A Study in Race Psychology,* trans. William A. White. New York, Journal of Nervous and Mental Disease Publishing Company, 1913.

——, "The Psycho-sexual Differences Between Hysteria and Dementia Praecox," in *Selected Papers on Psychoanalysis,* trans. Douglas Bryan and Alix Strachey. London, Hogarth Press, 1950; New York, Basic Books, 1953.

Ackerman, Nathan W., "Family Psychotherapy," *American Journal of Psychotherapy,* Vol. XX, No. 3 (July, 1966).

Althusser, Louis, "Freud et Lacan," *La Nouvelle Critique,* January, 1965.

Amado, Georges, "Douze Ans de pratique médico-pédagogique," in *La Psychiatrie de l'enfant,* Vol. IV. Paris, Presses Universitaires de France, 1961–62.

Anzieu, Didier, "Étude psychanalytique des groupes réels," *Les Temps modernes,* No. 242 (July, 1966).

Apley, John, and Ronald MacKeith, *The Child and His Symptoms.* Philadelphia, F. A. Davis; Oxford, Blackwell Scientific Publications, 1962.

Aubry, Jenny, *La Carence des soins maternels.* Paris, Éditions de la Parole, 1965. 1st ed.: Paris, Presses Universitaires de France, 1955.

———, "Médecine psychosomatique chez l'enfant du premier âge à l'hôpital," in *Médecine psychosomatique*. Paris, Expansion Scientifique Française, 1965.

———, "Pédiatrie psychosomatique à l'hôpital des enfants malades, service de J. Aubry," *Revue de médecine psychosomatique*, Vol. V, No. 4 (1963).

———, "La Relation du rééducateur du langage et de l'enfant," in *Relations affectives enfants-éducateurs*. Association Nationale des Centres Psycho-pédagogiques, day seminars, May 19–21, 1966.

———, and Raymonde Bargues, "Les Facteurs psychologiques de l'hospitalisation," in *Problèmes actuelles de pédiatrie*, Vol. IX. Basle and New York, Karger, 1965.

Aulagnier, Piera, "Essai d'approche d'une conception psychanalytique des psychoses," lectures at the Hôpital Sainte-Anne, 1964. Unpublished.

———, "Remarques sur la structure psychotique," *La Psychanalyse*, Vol. VIII (1963).

———, "Sur le concept d'identification," lectures at the Hôpital Sainte-Anne, 1964. Unpublished.

Binswanger, Ludwig, "The Case of Ellen West" (trans. W. M. Mendel and J. Lyons), "The Existential Analysis School of Thought" (trans. Ernest Angel), and "Insanity as Life-Historical Phenomenon and as Mental Disease" (trans. Angel), in Rollo May *et al.*, eds., *Existence —a New Dimension in Psychiatry and Psychology*. New York, Basic Books, 1958.

Bion, W. R., "Language and the Schizophrenic," in Melanie Klein *et al.*, eds., *New Directions in Psychoanalysis*. London, Tavistock, 1955; New York, Basic Books, 1956.

Bleuler, Eugen, *Dementia praecox oder Gruppe der Schizophrenien*. Leipzig and Vienna, Deuticke, 1911.

———, *Dementia Praecox or the Group of Schizophrenias*, trans. Joseph Zinkin. New York, International Universities Press, 1950; London, Allen & Unwin, 1951.

Bleuler, Manfred, "Eugen Bleuler's Conception of Schizophrenia, an Historical Sketch," *Bulletin of the Isaac Ray Medical Library* (Providence, R.I.), 1953.

Burlingham, Dorothy, *et al.*, "Simultaneous Analysis of Mother and

Child," in *The Psychoanalytic Study of the Child,* Vol. X. New York, International Universities Press; London, Imago, 1955.

Buxbaum, Edith, "Technique of Child Psychotherapy," in *The Psychoanalytic Study of the Child,* Vol. IX. New York, International Universities Press; London, Imago, 1954.

Castets, Bruno, "L'Enfant nounours," *Annales médico-psychologiques,* Vol. I, No. 5 (1967).

Diatkine, R., and C. Stein, "Les Psychoses de l'enfant," *Évolution psychiatrique,* No. 2 (1958).

Dolto, Françoise, "Hypothèses nouvelles concernant les réactions de jalousie à la naissance d'un puîné," *Psyché,* Nos. 7, 9, 10 (1947).

Erikson, Erik H., "A Neurological Crisis in a Small Boy: Sam," in *Childhood and Society,* 2nd ed. New York, Norton, 1964; London, Penguin Books, 1965.

——, "Childhood and Tradition in Two American Indian Tribes," in *The Psychoanalytic Study of the Child,* Vol. I. New York, International Universities Press; London, Imago, 1945.

Ey, Henri, *L'Inconscient.* Paris, Desclée de Brouwer, 1966.

Faergeman, Poul Martin, *Psychogenic Psychoses.* London, Butterworth, 1963.

Ferenczi, Sandor, "The Psychic Consequences of a Castration," in *Further Contributions to the Theory and Technique of Psychoanalysis,* trans. Jane Isabel Suttie *et al.,* comp. John Rickman. London, Hogarth Press, 1951; New York, Basic Books, 1952.

Foucault, Michel, *Madness and Civilization: A History of Insanity in the Age of Reason,* trans. Richard Howard. New York, Pantheon Books, 1965; London, Tavistock, 1967.

——, *The Order of Things,* trans. Alan Sheridan-Smith. New York, Pantheon Books; London, Tavistock, 1970.

Fraiberg, Selma H., "Clinical Notes on the Nature of Transference in Child Analysis," in *The Psychoanalytic Study of the Child,* Vol. VI. New York, International Universities Press; London, Imago, 1951.

Freud, Anna, *The Ego and the Mechanisms of Defense,* trans. Cecil Baines. New York, International Universities Press, 1948; London, Hogarth Press, 1954.

——, *The Psycho-analytical Treatment of Children,* trans. Nancy

Proctor-Gregg. London, Imago, 1946; 3rd ed.: New York, Anglo-books, 1951.

Freud, Sigmund, *Complete Psychological Works of Sigmund Freud* (Standard Edition), trans. and ed. James Strachey. London, Hogarth Press, 1966. 24 vols.

———, "Analysis of a Phobia in a Five-Year-Old Boy" (Little Hans), Vol. X.

———, *Beyond the Pleasure Principle,* Vol. XVIII.

———, "Dreams and Occultism" (No. 30 in *New Introductory Lectures on Psychoanalysis*), Vol. XXII.

———, "Fragment of Analysis of a Case of Hysteria" (Dora), Vol. VII.

———, "Further Remarks on the Defence Neuro-psychoses," Vol. III.

———, "History of an Infantile Neurosis" (Wolf Man), Vol. XVII.

———, *Mourning and Melancholia,* Vol. XIV.

———, "Notes upon a Case of Obsessional Neurosis" (Rat Man), Vol. X.

———, "On the History of the Psycho-analytical Movement," Vol. XIV.

———, *An Outline of Psychoanalysis,* Vol. XXI.

———, "The Poet and Daydreaming," Vol. IX.

———, "Preface to Aichhorn's *Wayward Youth,*" Vol. XIX.

———, *A General Selection from the Works of Sigmund Freud,* ed. John Rickman. London, Hogarth Press, 1937; New York, Doubleday Anchor Books, 1957.

———, *The Interpretation of Dreams,* trans. and ed. James Strachey. London, Allen & Unwin, 1954; New York, Basic Books, 1955.

———, *The Origins of Psycho-analysis: Letters to Wilhelm Fliess, Drafts and Notes, 1887–1902,* ed. Marie Bonaparte *et al.* New York, Basic Books, 1954.

Glover, Edward, "Examination of the Klein System of Child Psychology," in *The Psychoanalytic Study of the Child,* Vol. I. New York, International Universities Press; London, Imago, 1945.

Green, André, "L'Objet (a) de J. Lacan, sa logique, et la théorie freudienne," *Cahiers pour l'analyse,* No. 3 (May, 1966).

Grinberg, Léon, "Psicopatología de la identificación y contraidentificación proyectivas y de la contratrasferencia," *Revista de psicoanálisis* (Buenos Aires), Vol. XX, No. 2 (April–June, 1963).

Haworth, Mary R., ed., *Child Psychotherapy: Practice and Theory.* New York, Basic Books, 1964.

Hellman, Ilse, *et al.,* "Simultaneous Analysis of a Mother and Child," in *The Psychoanalytic Study of the Child,* Vol. XV. New York, International Universities Press; London, Imago, 1960.

Hesnard, Angelo L. M., *L'Oeuvre de Freud et son importance pour le monde moderne.* Paris, Payot, 1960.

Irigaray, Luce, "Communication linguistique et communication spéculaire," *Cahiers pour l'analyse,* No. 3 (May, 1966).

Itard, Jean, *The Wild Boy of Aveyron,* trans. George and Muriel Humphrey. New York and London, D. Appleton-Century, 1932.

Kanner, Leo, *Child Psychiatry.* Springfield, Ill., Charles C Thomas, 1935; London, Baillière, Tindall & Cox, 1936.

Klein, Melanie, "Mourning and Its Relation to Manic-Depressive States," in *Contributions to Psychoanalysis, 1921–1945.* London, Hogarth Press, 1948; New York, Anglobooks, 1952.

——, "Notes on Some Schizoid Mechanisms," in Melanie Klein *et al., Developments in Psychoanalysis,* ed. Joan Riviere. London, Hogarth Press, 1952.

——, "The Oedipus Complex in the Light of Early Anxieties," in *Contributions to Psychoanalysis, 1921–1945.* London, Hogarth Press, 1948; New York, Anglobooks, 1952.

——, "Les Origines du transfert," *Revue française de psychanalyse,* Vol. XVI, No. 1 (January, 1952).

——, *Our Adult World and Other Essays,* ed. Elliot Jaques and Betty Joseph. New York, Basic Books; London, Heinemann, 1963. (British title: *Our Adult Medical World and Other Essays.*)

——, *The Psychoanalysis of Children.* New York, Norton; London, Hogarth Press, 1932.

——, "The Psychotherapy of the Psychoses," in *Contributions to Psychoanalysis, 1921–1945.* London, Hogarth Press, 1948; New York, Anglobooks, 1952.

——, Paula Heimann, and R. E. Money-Kyrle, eds., *New Directions in Psychoanalysis.* London, Tavistock, 1955; New York, Basic Books, 1956.

Kraepelin, Emil, *Psychiatrie,* 5th ed. Leipzig, Barth, 1896.

Kut, Sara, "The Changing Patterns of Transference in the Analysis of an Eleven-Year-Old Girl," in *The Psychoanalytic Study of the Child,* Vol. VIII. New York, International Universities Press; London, Imago, 1953.

Lacan, Jacques, "Le Désir et son interprétation," *Bulletin de psychologie,* Vol. XIII, Nos. 5–6 (January, 1960). Seminars of November, 1958–February, 1959; report by J.-B. Pontalis.

———, "La Direction de la cure et les principes de son pouvoir," in *Écrits.* Paris, Éditions du Seuil, 1966.

———, "La Famille," in *La Vie mentale,* Vol. VIII of the *Encyclopédie française,* ed. A. de Monzie. Paris, Société de Gestion de l'Encyclopédie Française, 1938.

———, "Fonction et champ de la parole et du langage en psychanalyse," in *Écrits.* Paris, Éditions du Seuil, 1966.

———, "Les Formations de l'inconscient," *Bulletin de psychologie,* Vol. XII, Nos. 2–4 (November–December, 1958). Seminars of November, 1957–June, 1958; report by J.-B. Pontalis.

———, "Intervention sur le transfert," *Revue française de psychanalyse,* Vol. XVI, Nos. 1–2 (1952). Intervention at the Congrès de Psychanalystes de Langue Romaine. (Reprinted in *Écrits.* Paris, Éditions du Seuil, 1966.)

———, "Position de l'inconscient," in *Écrits.* Paris, Éditions du Seuil, 1966.

———, "Propos sur la causalité psychique," in *Écrits.* Paris, Éditions du Seuil, 1966.

———, "D'une question préliminaire à tout traitement possible de la psychose," in *Écrits.* Paris, Éditions du Seuil, 1966.

———, "La Relation d'objet et les structures freudiennes," *Bulletin de psychologie,* Vol. X, Nos. 7, 10, 12, 14 (April–June, 1957); Vol. XI, No. 1 (September, 1957). Seminars of November, 1956–September, 1957; report by J.-B. Pontalis.

———, "La Science et la vérité," in *Écrits.* Paris, Éditions du Seuil, 1966.

———, "Situation de la psychanalyse en 1956," in *Écrits.* Paris, Éditions du Seuil, 1966.

————, "Du traitement possible de la psychose," in *Écrits*. Paris, Éditions du Seuil, 1966.

Laing, R. D., *The Divided Self*. London, Tavistock, 1960, 1969; New York, Pantheon Books, 1969.

————, *Self and Others*. London, Tavistock, 1961, 1969; New York, Pantheon Books, 1969.

———— and Aaron Esterson, *Sanity, Madness and the Family*. London, Tavistock, 1964; New York, Basic Books, 1965.

Lang, J.-L., "L'Abord psychanalytique des psychoses chez l'enfant," *La Psychanalyse*, Vol. IV (1958).

Laplanche, Jean, and Serge Leclaire, "L'Inconscient," *Les Temps modernes,* No. 183 (July, 1961).

Lebovici, Serge, and Joyce McDougall, *Un Cas de psychose infantile*. Paris, Presses Universitaires de France, 1960. (A revision and translation by Joyce McDougall, *Dialogue with Sammy: A Psychoanalytical Contribution to the Understanding of Child Psychosis,* was published in 1969 by the Hogarth Press, London.)

Leclaire, Serge, "A la recherche des principes d'une psychothérapie des psychoses," *Évolution psychiatrique,* April, 1958.

Malson, Lucien, *Les Enfants sauvages, mythe et réalité, suivi de Mémoire et rapport sur Victor de l'Aveyron, par Jean Itard*. Paris, Union Générale d'Éditions, 1964.

Mannoni, Maud, "Problèmes posés par la psychothérapie des débiles," *Sauvegarde de l'enfance,* January, 1965.

Mannoni, Octave, "Rêve et transfert," *La Psychanalyse,* Vol. VIII (1963).

————, "Je sais bien . . . mais quand même," *Les Temps modernes,* No. 212 (January, 1964).

————, "Itard et son sauvage," *Les Temps modernes,* No. 233 (October, 1965).

Oury, Fernand, and Aïda Vasquez, *Vers une pédagogie institutionnelle*. Paris, F. Maspero, 1967.

Pichon-Rivière, A.-A., "Quelques Considérations sur le transfert et contretransfert dans la psychanalyse d'enfants," *Revue française de psychanalyse,* Vol. XVI, Nos. 1–2 (January–June, 1952).

Rodriguez, Emilio, "The Analysis of a Three-Year-Old Mute Schizophrenic," in Melanie Klein *et al.,* eds., *New Directions in Psy-*

choanalysis. London, Tavistock, 1955; New York, Basic Books, 1956.

Rosenfeld, Herbert, "Notes on the Psychoanalysis of the Superego Conflict in an Acute Schizophrenic Patient," in Melanie Klein *et al.,* eds., *New Directions in Psychoanalysis.* London, Tavistock, 1955; New York, Basic Books, 1956.

Rosolato, Guy, and Daniel Widlocher, "Karl Abraham: Lecture de son oeuvre," *La Psychanalyse,* Vol. IV (1958).

Safouan, M., "Le Phallus dans le rapport mère-enfant." Unpublished.

Séchehaye, Marguerite A., *A New Psychotherapy in Schizophrenia,* trans. Grace Rubin-Rabson. New York, Grune & Stratton, 1956.

Shakow, David, and David Rapaport, *The Influence of Freud on American Psychology.* New York, International Universities Press, 1964.

Smirnoff, Victor, "Un Certain Savoir ou quelques propos sur le 11e congrès international de psychiatrie" (Zurich, 1957), *La Psychanalyse,* Vol. IV (1958).

Stanton, Alfred H., and Morris S. Schwartz, *The Mental Hospital.* New York, Basic Books; London, Tavistock, 1954.

Stern, A.-L., "Qu'est-ce qui fait consulter pour un enfant?" in *Relations affectives enfants-éducateurs.* Association Nationale des Centres Psycho-pédagogiques, day seminars, May 19–21, 1966.

Strauss, A., *et al., Psychiatric Ideologies and Institutions.* New York, Free Press; London, Macmillan, 1964.

"Symposium on Child Analysis," *International Journal of Psychoanalysis,* Vol. VIII (1927). Symposium held before the British Psycho-analytical Society, London, May 18–19, 1927.

Szasz, Thomas S., *The Myth of Mental Illness: Foundations of a Theory of Personal Conduct.* New York, Hoeber-Harper, 1961; London, Secker & Warburg, 1962.

——, "Psychiatry in Public Schools," *Teachers College Record* (Columbia University, New York), Vol. LXVI, No. 1 (1964).

Tosquelles, François, "Introduction au problème du transfert en psychothérapie institutionnelle," *Revue de psychothérapie institutionnelle,* No. 1.

——, "Pédagogie et psychothérapie institutionnelles," *Revue de psychothérapie institutionnelle,* Nos. 2–3.

————, *Pratique du maternage thérapeutique chez les débiles mentaux profonds*. Paris, Jean-Louis Aupetit, 1966.

Valabrega, Jean-Paul, "Aux sources de la psychanalyse," *Critique,* May, 1956.

Waelhans, Alphonse de, "Crise de la psychanalyse," *Critique,* March, 1958.

Winnicott, D. W., "Psychoanalysis and the Sense of Guilt," in *The Maturational Processes and the Facilitating Environment.* New York, International Universities Press; London, Hogarth Press, 1965.

Woltmann, Adolf G., "Varieties of Play Techniques," in Mary R. Haworth, ed., *Child Psychotherapy: Practice and Theory.* New York, Basic Books, 1964.

NOTE AND GLOSSARY
ON LACANIAN TERMINOLOGY

I have been asked to comment on the usage in this book of certain key terms that were coined originally by Jacques Lacan, whose works are not likely to be familiar to readers of the English translation. These terms do not lend themselves readily to translation, yet many were successfully rendered into English by Anthony Wilden in his book on Lacan, *The Language of the Self*. As Wilden's translations and expositions of Lacanian terms could hardly be improved upon, I have used a number of them to make up this glossary. Readers with further interest in the subject will want to turn to Wilden's book.

The present work owes much to the fact that Lacan offers a fresh orientation toward the understanding of Freudian discoveries. My comments are not to be construed as even a partial exposition of Lacan's work, but some acquaintance with it is certain to make the reading of this book easier.

Fundamentally, Lacan's goal is to return to Freud; it is his view that we have strayed from him. Rather than presuming to amend or perfect Freudian doctrines, Lacan claims that they have been allowed to degenerate; consequently, he returns to the literal interpretation of the texts. He shows us how the techniques of dream interpretation teach us to decipher the unconscious by treating it as a language. Dream images must not be treated as pictures of objects or as signs designating objects but, to use a linguistic term, as *signifiers,* like pieces of a jigsaw puzzle. The meaning is not to be searched for in some symbolistic conception

such as Jung has charted; it lies in the interrelationship of the signifiers. Freud anticipated the discoveries of de Saussure before the science
of linguistics had developed its methodology.

Nevertheless, Lacan's formulation, "The unconscious is structured
like a language," was surprising when he first posed it. Needless to say,
a variety of conclusions were drawn from it. For example, there were
those who ended up believing that the unconscious is a reservoir of
drives and instincts, serving as the intermediary between biology and
psychology. But when Freud showed us that the unconscious speaks,
although its language is different from that of conscious speech, it
was to compel us to abandon any attempt to base psychoanalysis on
biological foundations, such as the dynamics of instinct. Another conclusion was that the self is not the subject of the word; it is no longer
the "self" that was posited in Freud's early work that reconciled the
demands of the id with those of reality, but the self in the sense of narcissism.

Since 1936, having established the importance of what he called the
mirror-stage, Lacan has been pointing out the *Imaginary* origin of the
self. He demonstrated thereby the speculative origin of aggressivity—a
concept sketched out in his doctoral dissertation and revived in 1932.
The dissertation dealt with paranoiac psychosis, and in fact he derived
his theories from clinical observations of psychosis. Lacan's formulations have evolved from these foundations over a period of thirty years,
and it is clearly not possible to summarize them here. Suffice it to say
that in his collected *Écrits* Lacan's writings are unmarred by discrepan-
cies, despite the widely separated dates of their origin.

Lacan's work as a clinician is well known to those who have worked
with him in one capacity or another, or those who have been analyzed
by him, yet he has written almost nothing about it. He has devoted his
interest entirely to theory.

It can safely be said that Lacan's concerns have focused on the relationship between subject and language. He claims that language precedes the formation of the subject's image and can be said to engender
it. For example, the infant has a place in parental discourse before he

is born; he has a name; he will be "spoken" as long as he is the object of care; the neglect of his needs—to which we sometimes attach so much importance, as in regard to frustrations—will have far less effect on him than the nature and the "accidents" of discourse that surround him. The specifically human environment is neither biological nor social, but linguistic.

Lacan's ideas had been widely disseminated even before their publication. They had influenced researchers in other disciplines, and they also coincided with the findings of independent scholars.

The publication of his *Écrits* in 1966 created the impression that Lacan was joining the antihumanist movement spearheaded by Claude Lévi-Strauss and Michel Foucault, but the dates of his texts alone should have dispelled that delusion.

Lacan's work is not easily grasped; it is difficult to read and still more difficult to translate. Nevertheless, those who delve into it find the cause of difficulty in his precision, above all, and not in the obscure style, as is so readily believed. This is not to say that the style is unimportant, for Lacan takes advantage of every means that offers a better approach to unconscious thought, means that not even Freud employed although he described them, for example in his book on wit. The uninitiated reader will be amazed at encountering puns in such a serious work and put off by coming across an absurd parallel, but Lacan regards this style, and particularly the systematic usage of ellipses, as necessary in the training of analysts, because it facilitates access to the unconscious.

At the present time, we are witnessing a drastic revision of intellectual positions in France, sweeping across a vast range of disciplines from literature to ethnography. It is quite likely that certain aspects of this ferment are but vagaries of fashion, but only certain ones, whereas others appear to have made lasting advances. Should "Lacanism" be carried forward by this trend and momentarily benefit from it, the gain will be more apparent than real, for Lacan's theories are solidly rooted in Freud's own texts and their fate is by no means linked to the evolution of a particular trend. His opponents, analysts who are against him for ideological reasons, remain for the most part interested in his theoretical work and often follow it with keen attention. It is un-doubtedly necessary to extract, revise, and especially to elucidate; but just as undoubtedly, Lacan's imprint on psychoanalysis will not vanish with changing fashions. His work is gradually becoming known outside France, although time will have to pass before its meaning can be solidly grasped.

The following glossary is composed of quotations from Anthony Wilden's translation of and commentary on Jacques Lacan's "Discours de Rome," *The Language of the Self: The Function of Language in Psychoanalysis* (Baltimore, The Johns Hopkins Press, 1968). The page numbers in brackets under the key words refer to Wilden's text. Source notes in brackets following the quotations from Lacan refer to Lacan's published works in French.

ANXIETY (*angoisse*)
[p. 150]
Both the Freudian and the Heideggerian *Angst* have been generally trans-lated "anxiety" in English, "angoisse" in French. But Freud, unlike Heideg-ger, by no means uses this term, sanctified since "existentialism," in an en-tirely coherent way, although he does stress the anticipatory element and the absence of an object in *Angst,* as Heidegger does. . . .

In the seminar of May–July, 1957, on "La Relation d'objet et les structures freudiennes," speaking in relation to little Hans, Lacan defined "angoisse" as follows: *"Angoisse* is not the fear of an object, but the confrontation of the subject with an absence of object, with a lack of being in which he is stuck or caught, in which he loses himself and to which anything is preferable, even the forging of that most strange and alien of objects: a phobia."

DESIRE (*désir*)
[p. 114]
In 1946 Lacan paraphrased Hegel as follows:

The very desire of man, [Hegel] tells us, is constituted under the sign of mediation; it is desire to make its desire recognized. It has for its object a desire, that of the other, in the sense that there is no object for man's desire which is constituted without some sort of mediation—which appears in his most primitive needs: for example, even his food has to be prepared—and which is found again throughout the development of satisfaction from the moment of the master-slave conflict throughout the dialectic of labor. ["Propos sur la causalité psychique," *Écrits*, p. 151.]

In the "Direction de la cure" (1961), Lacan summarizes his remarks on the nature of desire:

> One of the principles which follows these premises is that:
> —if desire is an effect in the subject of that condition which is imposed on him by the existence of the discourse, to make his need pass through the defiles of the signifier;
> —if on the other hand . . . , by opening up the dialectic of transference, we must ground the notion of the Other with a big O as being the locus of the deployment of the Word (the other scene, *eine andere Schauplatz*, of which Freud speaks in the *Traumdeutung*);
> —it must be posited that, as a facet of an animal at the mercy of Language, man's desire is desire of the Other.
> This formulation is aimed at quite another function than that of the primary identification mentioned earlier in this article, for it is not a question of the assumption by the subject of the *insignia* of the other, but rather the condition that the subject has to find the constituting structure of his desire in the same *béance* opened up by the effect of the signifiers in those who come [through transference] to represent the Other for him, insofar as his demand is subjected to them. ["La direction de la cure et les principes de son pouvoir," *Écrits*, p. 585.]

DISCOURSE, LANGUAGE *(discours, langage)*
[p. 122]

> "What link do you make," I heard myself asked, "between that instrument of Language, whose given data man must accept every bit as much as those of the Real, and that grounding function which you say is the function of the Word insofar as it constitutes the subject in an intersubjective relation?"
> I reply: in making Language the intermediary in which to set the analytic experience to rights, it is not the sense of means implied by this term that I emphasize, but that of locus. . . .
> I add that it is from the point of view of the notion of communication that I deliberately orient my conception of Language; its function as expression, as far as I know, was mentioned only once in my report.
> Let me therefore say precisely what Language signifies in what it communicates: it is neither signal, nor sign, nor even sign of the thing insofar as the thing is an exterior reality. The relation between signifier and signified is entirely enclosed in the order of Language itself, which completely conditions its two terms.
> Let us examine the term signifier first of all. It is constituted by a set

of material elements linked by a structure of which I shall indicate presently the extent to which it is simple in its elements, or even where one can situate its point of origin. But, even if I have to pass for a materialist, it is on the fact that it is a question of material that I shall insist first of all, and in order to emphasize, in this question of locus which we are discussing, the place occupied by this material. This is with the sole purpose of destroying the mirage which by a process of elimination seems to assign to the human brain the locus of the phenomenon of language. Well, where could it be then? Replying for the signifier: "everywhere else." [Lacan then mentions modern communication theory which has given to the reduction of the signifier into nonsignifying units (Hartley units) the "scientific" status of use in industry, and then to the "frozen words" of Rabelais, which anticipate the "two pounds or so of signifier" rolled up in the recorder in front of him.]

Let us move on to the signified. If it is not the thing, as I told you, what is it then? Precisely the sense. The discourse which I am delivering to you here . . . is concerned with an experience common to all of us, but you will estimate its value insofar as it communicates to you the sense of that experience, and not the experience itself. . . .

And this sense, where is it? The correct reply here, "nowhere," if opposed—when it is a question of the signified—to the correct reply that suited the signifier, will not disappoint my questioner any the less, if he expected in it something approaching the "denomination of things." For, besides the fact that no "part of speech" has the privilege of such a function, contrary to the grammatical appearances which attribute this function to the substantive, meaning is never capable of being sensed except in the uniqueness of the signification developed by the discourse.

Thus it is that interhuman communication is always information on information, put to the test of a community of Language, a numbering and a perfecting of the target which will surround the objects, themselves born of the concurrence of a primordial rivalry.

No doubt that the discourse is concerned with things. It is in fact in this encounter that from realities they become things. It is so true that the word is not the sign of the thing, that the word tends to become the thing itself. But it is only insofar as it abandons the sense. . . .

If someone should oppose me with the traditional view that it is the definition that gives the word its meaning, I would not say no: after all it was not I who said that every word presupposes by its use the entire discourse of the dictionary . . . —or even that of all the texts of a given language. [Lacan, "Fonction et champ de la parole et du langage en psychanalyse," *Écrits*, p. 237–323.]

IDENTIFICATION (*identification*)
[pp. 294, 295, 296]

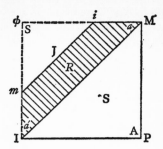

SCHÉMA R:

KEY

S	the subject
I	the Imaginary (at upper left)
R	the Real (shaded area)
S	the Symbolic (at lower right)
a	the figure of the Imaginary other of the *stade du miroir*
a'	the identification of the (child's) ego through the identification with the ideal of the ego (the paternal *imago*)
ϕ	the phallus (Imaginary object)
I	the ideal of the ego
P	the position of the Name-of-the-Father in the locus of the Other
M	the signifier of the primordial object (*das Ding*—cf. Freud on negation) —the mother, who is the *real Other*.
i }	the two Imaginary end-points of all later narcissistic relationships,
m }	the ego (*m*) and the specular image (*i*).
iM	the axis of desires (object choice)
mI	the axis of identifications (narcissism)
SA	the *metaphorical* relationship between the subject and the Other or between the phallus (ϕ) and the Name-of-the-Father (P)—cf. Schema L.

The broken line delimits the Imaginary.

Beginning from the position of the (child) subject—identified as in classical analytical theory with the phallus—one notes the two lines of interest which link him to the ideal of the ego (I) and the signifier (M) of the real Other, the mother. The first represents the nonsexual relationship of identification with an ideal (being the other) . . . the second, the libidinal relationship of desire for the mother as an object (having the other). At the same time the primordial triangle of father-child-mother represented as I-S(ϕ)-M is given at a secondary level (*m-S-i*) representing all the later identifications, narcissistic relationships, and Imaginary captures in which the subject may be involved. The solid line joining *i* and M represents the *real* relationship between the child and the primordial object (the mother or a part of her body) at a time when the child cannot distinguish himself from "reality." This is of course in keeping both with Freud's remarks, previously referred to, in the article on the *Verneinung* as well as with Lacan's view of the Real as outside symbolization, since for the mother to symbolize "reality" she must become a signifier in the Symbolic for the subject, introjection and expulsion being neither Real nor Imaginary. On the other hand, the relationship between ego (*m*) and the ideal of the ego (I) is shown as a broken line; it is always Imaginary. Thus the distance between *m* and I and that between *i* and M represent the distinction the subject has achieved between the primordial relationships of being and having (I and M) and later ones; this delimits the Real for the subject. In psychosis this delimitation becomes warped or twisted. The Real and the Imaginary are represented more closely related to each other than is each to the Symbolic, Lacan's intention presumably being to assert the primacy of the Symbolic over both, since they derive their structure from it (the signifier precedes and determines the signified).

The *objectal* movement of the subject's desire toward the mother is complemented by the mother's desire. Her desire (the desire of the Other) that he *be* the phallus (the signifier of the desire of the Other) so that she may have it is met by the child's desire to conform to her desire (to be what his mother wants him to be)—in the Lacanian view the neurotic or psychotic subject has to learn that this is what he wants to be and precisely what he cannot be. The *identificatory* movement towards the ideal is a pure alienation along the lines of the *stade du miroir,* but again the subject meets a contrary law: his desire to be the father (in the father's place) complements the rivalry which his relationship to the mother also sets up. Naturally the respective lines of interest represent any number of intermediate positions, whether from the static or the historical point of view.

The Name-of-the-Father in this formulation means rather precisely what it says. P represents the Word of the father as employed by the mother—in other words, it represents the authority of the father upon which she calls in her dealings with the child. Thus is the Symbolic father the figure of the Law to which the real or Imaginary father may or may not conform. The anaclitic and primary relationship of the child to the mother is mediated by the "object *a*" (apparently complemented in the relationship to the *imago* of the father by its image in *a'*). Originally the child is involved in an identification with another springing from his identification with objects at a stage where he does not distinguish between object love and identification love; it is at this point, in Lacan's view, that the progressive splitting of demand from need and the resulting birth of desire occur. It is at this point—structurally speaking—that the mother introduces into the child's view of "reality" the fact of the lack of object upon which desire depends. This lack of object is an absence; the Imaginary other (*a*) is now only a substitute for it, since a lack cannot be "specularized." . . . Weaning, for instance, sometimes described in psychoanalysis as a primordial form of castration—inaccurately it seems, since the "castration" of the "castration complex" is not and cannot be real—is an especially significant discovery of absence for the child. With the constitution of the lack of object, need gives rise to demand and desire.

IMAGINARY, SYMBOLIC, REAL (*imaginaire, symbolique, réel*)
[p. 92]
Le symbolique, l'imaginaire, and *le réel* are the three "orders"—basically, the discursive, the perceptive, and the real orders—introduced into psycho-analytical terminology by Lacan in 1953.

For some remarks on the Imaginary and its relation to the Symbolic and the Real, see the 1958 article by Leclaire on psychosis. ["A la recherche d'une psychothérapie des psychoses," *L'Évolution psychiatrique,* 1958, pp. 377–411.] Leclaire says in part: "The experience of the Real presupposes the simultaneous use of two correlative functions, the Imaginary function and the Symbolic function. That is Imaginary which, like shadows, has no existence of its own, and yet whose absence, in the light of life, cannot be conceived; that which, without power of distinction inundates singularity and thus escapes any truly rational grasp. That is Imaginary which is irremediably opposed or which is indistinctly confused, without any dialectical movement; the dream is Imaginary . . . just as long as it is not interpreted." And later: "no symbol can do without Imaginary support."

The topographical regression of the "dream thoughts" to images in the dream might be described as a process of the Symbolic becoming Imaginary. [p. 161]
Since the Symbolic, the Imaginary, and the Real co-exist and intersect in the subject—the Real is not synonymous with external reality, but rather with what is real for the subject—at the same time as they are functions linking the subject to others and to the world, any change in one order will have repercussions on the others. The Symbolic is the primary order, since it represents and structures both of the others; moreover, since it is ultimately only in language (or in judgment) that synonyms, ambiguities, and interpretations operate, Lacan avers that it is not possible to view the Freudian concept of overdetermination (of the symptom) as originating outside the Symbolic order.

LACK (*manque*)
[p. 218]
. . . Lacan's notion of a primordial "lack" is precisely the "lack of a fixed point" (the impossibility for desire to recover the lost object) toward which

desire and consequently the metonymic movement of discourse is aimed. It is a lack providing for the absent center (the object) and is thus simply a reversal of the fixed point. Lacan's view does not seem to dispense with the transcendental referent presupposed in psychoanalysis: for him this referent is the lost object at the origins. The system is set in motion by the mechanisms generated by the passage from need to desire through demand. Presence becomes absence—and no substitute in the system of substitutions is ever adequate to its object.

LANGUAGE (*langage*): see DISCOURSE

LAW (*loi*)
[p. 270]
The symbolic has wider connotations also. In another sense it is exactly equivalent to Lévi-Strauss's notion of the "world of rules" and the "symbolic relationships" into which we are born and to which we learn to conform, however much our dreams may express our wish for a disorder or a counter-order. The "familial constellation" into which we arrive as strangers to humanity is already part of it. The Symbolic is the unconscious order for Lacan, just as it is for Lévi-Strauss, however divergent their intentions. Thus it designates a symbolic structure based on a linguistic model composed of chains of signifiers (some of which, however—the somatic symptoms, for instance—are in fact signs). And in the same way that Lévi-Strauss's concept of the "symbolic function" in human society depends upon the *law* which founds society (the law of incest), so Lacan's notion of the Symbolic order depends upon the law of the father. This is his notion of the Symbolic Father, or what he calls the Name-of-the-Father—that is, a signifier in a linguistic model—which is related to his theory of psychosis.

ME, I (*moi, je*)
[p. 101]
There is a nice distinction between the ego-ideal and the ideal-ego, a distinction never methodologically clarified by Freud, and Lacan's assimilation of narcissism to identification is in the tradition of that same ambiguity. At the same time, Lacan's use of *moi* shares the *Ich*'s sense of "self," as Freud sometimes employs it, especially in the earlier works.

> The concept of the *moi* which Freud demonstrated particularly in the theory of narcissism viewed as the source of all enamoration or "falling in love" (*Verliebtheit*)—and in the technique of resistance viewed as supported by the latent and patent forms of *dénégation* (*Verneinung*)—

brings out in the most precise way its function of irreality: mirage and misconstruction. He completed the concept by a genetic view which situates the *moi* clearly in the order of the Imaginary relations and which shows in its radical alienation the matrix which specifies interhuman aggressivity as essentially intrasubjective. ["Fonction et champ de la parole et du langage en psychanalyse," *Écrits*, pp. 237–323.]

[p. 147]
Now the Real confronted by analysis is a man who must be allowed to go on speaking. It is in proportion to the sense that the subject effectively brings to pronouncing the *"je"* which decides whether he is or is not *the one who is speaking*. [*Ibid.*]

METAPHOR OF THE FATHER (*métaphore paternelle*)
[pp. 270–1]
The Symbolic father is not a real or an Imaginary father (*imago*), but corresponds to the mythical Symbolic father of *Totem and Taboo*. The requirements of Freud's theory, says Lacan, led him "to link the apparition of the signifier of the Father, as author of the Law, to death, or rather to the murder of the Father, thus demonstrating that if this murder is the fruitful moment of the debt through which the subject binds himself for life to the Law, the Symbolic Father, insofar as he signifies that Law, is actually the dead Father." This primal of all primal scenes is related in Freud to the "primal repression," for which Lacan substitutes the terms "constituting metaphor" or "paternal metaphor." It is through the failure of this paternal metaphor, according to Lacan, that the psychotic is induced to foreclude (*verwerfen*) the Name-of-the-Father. Since the Name-of-the-Father has never been successfully repressed, it is rejected, and with it, asserts Lacan, the whole Symbolic order. If the subject employs figures of speech and metaphors in his delusions, it is because the signifier and the signified have coalesced for him to the point that he cannot tell symbol from the thing symbolized, or word from thing presentation. In some respects his discourse may resemble what linguists call autonomous messages, that is to say, messages about words rather than messages employing words. But eventually he will lose all his metalinguistic capacities, or so it will seem from outside.

MIRROR-STAGE (*stade du miroir*)
[p. 172]
In speaking of the relationship of aggressivity and narcissism, the one being correlative to the other, Lacan views the *stade du miroir* as the primary identification allowing the possibility of the secondary identification described by Freud as part of the function of the Oedipus relationship. . . . Thus aggressivity, for Lacan, is primarily intrasubjective. But is the

infans of the *stade du miroir* a subject? Lacan employs the term with a fine distinction: the child is a subject, he says, because, unlike the chimpanzee before a mirror, he recognizes what he sees and celebrates his discovery. But he is an alienated subject (a *moi*) by this very fact. His "true" subjectivity, as I interpret it, is only "restored" to him "in the universal" (that is, in the world of language) by his learning to speak.

The *stade du miroir* is further the "crossroads" through which the child is introduced to human desire.

NAME OF THE FATHER (*nom du père*)
[p. 126]

What is meant by *le nom du père* is elaborated in [Lacan's] later theoretical article on psychosis [1958, "D'une question préliminaire à tout traitement possible de la psychose," *Écrits*, pp. 531–85.] "The name of the father" is the signifier of "the function of the father," and the question of the sense in which these terms are to be taken is briefly dealt with in "La Psychanalyse et son enseignement" [*Écrits*, pp. 437–59]. The signifier is not only "to be taken *au pied de la lettre*, it *is* the letter."

NEED, DEMAND, DESIRE (*besoin, demande, désir*)
[p. 143]

The relation of *need, demand,* and *desire* and the relation of desire to the signifier are elaborated throughout the later writings of Lacan, and in detail in the unpublished seminars (see the summaries of J.-B. Pontalis): "It must be granted that it is the concrete incidence of the signifier in the submission of need to demand which, by repressing desire into the position of being faultily recognized, confers on the unconscious its order." ["A la mémoire d'Ernest Jones: Sur sa théorie du symbolisme," *La Psychanalyse,* Vol. V (January–March 1959), pp. 1–20.]

[p. 185]

The distinction between need, demand, and desire is an important aspect of Lacan's theory and the distinction is related to the Imaginary order.

The *parole vide* is an Imaginary discourse, a discourse impregnated with Imaginary elements which have to be resolved if the subject and analyst are to progress to the ideal point of the *parole pleine*. For Lacan, the main features of this Imaginary discourse are the demands (intransitive in fact) which the subject makes of the analyst. Desire, for him, on the other hand, is "an effect in the subject of that condition which is imposed upon him by the existence of the discourse to cause his need to pass through the defiles of the signifier." This is in effect an important and radical restatement in a structural terminology of the essentially genetic view of the subordination of the pleasure principle to the reality principle, since reality for the subject is literally *re-presented* by the signifier.

OBJECT (*objet*)
[p. 186]

Lacan's views on the relationship between the Symbolic, the Imaginary, and the Real, and their relationship to the phallus and to what is called the object relation in psychoanalysis are developed at length in the seminars on "La Relation d'objet et les structures freudiennes" [*Bulletin de psychologie*, 1956], but since these seminars depend on a lengthy structural analysis of a number of case histories, it is not possible to go into the details here. Lacan's main point is that traditional psychoanalysis has so concerned itself with the "reduced" dialectic of the subject and his relation to objects conceived of by analysts as either imaginary (hallucinated) or real, that the most essential part of the object relation has been ignored: the notion of the lack of object. Analysts have forgotten that "between the mother and the child, Freud introduced a third term, an Imaginary element, whose signifying role is a major one: the phallus" (Seminar of November–December, 1956, p. 427). This relationship of three terms, mother, child, and phallus, is changed through the function of the father, which "inserts the lack of object into a new dialectic" and provides for what psychoanalysis calls the "normalization" of the Oedipus complex. But the father involved is not the real father, or an *imago* of any real father—he is what Lacan calls the "Symbolic father."
[pp. 162–63]

What is especially important in the development of [Lacan's] views is the notion of the "partial object," derived from English psychoanalysis. Whereas Lacan says little about the object relation in the earlier works which is not a restatement in psychoanalytical terms of the Hegelian theory of desire, the growing emphasis in the later works is upon a reinterpretation of the Kleinian theories about the object relation. Thus there is a significant difference in the nature of the object involved: in the early works it is *"l'autre (petit a)"*; in the later ones it is *"l'objet a,"* which is a much more primordial relationship, a relationship to objects which is anterior to the child's relationship to a person as an object.

OTHER (*autre*)
[pp. 106–7]

The following passages from his later writings will be of assistance in clarifying Lacan's elaboration of this concept. In opposition to what he calls a certain "phenomenological" trend in psychoanalysis, Lacan refers to the divergence between himself and his colleague Daniel Lagache in the following terms:

> [Our divergence] lies in the actual function which he confers on intersubjectivity. For intersubjectivity is defined for him in a relation to the other [ness] of the counterpart [*l'autre du semblable*], a symmetrical relation in principle, as can be seen from the fact that Daniel Lagache sets up the formula that the subject learns to treat himself as an object through the other. My position is that the subject has to emerge from the given of the signifiers which cover him in an Other which is their transcendental locus: through this he constitutes himself in an existence where the manifestly constituting vector of the Freudian area of experience is possible: that is to say, what is called desire. ["Remarque sur le rapport de Daniel Lagache," *Écrits*, p. 64].

In the article on Merleau-Ponty in *Les Temps Modernes* (1961), Lacan points out the problematic involved in philosophizing from the primacy of the *cogito,* or from that of the *percipio:*

> To put it in a nutshell, it seems to me that the "I think" to which it is intended that presence be reduced, continues to imply, no matter how indeterminate one may make it, all the powers of the reflection [*réflexion*] by which subject and consciousness are confounded—namely, the mirage which psychoanalytic experience places at the basis [*principe*] of the *méconnaissance* of the subject and which I myself have tried to focus on in the *stade du miroir* by concentrating it there. ["Maurice Merleau-Ponty," *Les Temps Modernes*, Nos. 184–85 (1961), pp. 248–49.]

The structure of intersubjectivity is further elaborated as follows:

> Thus it is that if man comes to thinking the Symbolic order, it is because he is caught in it from the first in his being. The illusion that he has formed it by his consciousness results from the fact that it was by the way of a *béance* specific to his Imaginary relation to his counterpart, that he was able to enter into this order as a subject. But he was only able to make this entrance by the radical defile of the Word, the same, in fact, of which we have recognized a genetic moment in the play of the child [The *Fort! Da!* of *Beyond the Pleasure Principle*] but which, in its complete form, is reproduced each time that the subject addresses himself to the Other as absolute, that is to say, as the Other who can nullify the subject himself, in the same way as he can do for him, that is, by making himself an object in order to deceive him. This dialectic of intersubjectivity whose use I have shown to be necessary—from the theory of transference to the structure of paranoia itself—during the past three years of my seminar at Sainte-Anne, is readily backed up by the following schema which has long been familiar to my students:

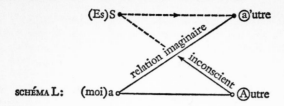

sᴄʜᴇ́ᴍᴀ L: (moi)a

The two middle terms represent the coupled reciprocal Imaginary objectification which I have emphasized in the *stade du miroir*. ["Le séminaire sur *La lettre volée*," *Écrits*, p. 11.]

There is a simplified and slightly different version of the schema in the "Traitement possible de la psychose" [*Écrits*, p. 531], with the following comments:

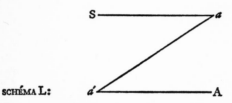

sᴄʜᴇ́ᴍᴀ L:

This schema signifies that the condition of the subject S (neurotic or psychotic) depends on what is being unfolded in the Other A. What is being unfolded there is articulated like a discourse (the unconscious the discourse of the Other)—a discourse whose syntax Freud first sought to define for those fragments of it which come to us in certain privileged moments, dreams, slips of the tongue or pen, flashes of wit.

How would the subject be an interested party in the discourse if he were not taking part? He is one, in fact, in that he is drawn to the four corners of the schema, which are: *S*, his ineffable and stupid existence; *a*, his objects, *á*, his *moi*—that is, what is reflected of his form in his objects; and *A*, the locus from which the question of his existence may put to him.

PHALLUS (*phallus*)
[p. 187]
Why speak of the phallus and not of the penis? Lacan asks.

. . . Because the phallus is not a question of a form, or of an image, or of a phantasy, but rather of a signifier, the signifier of desire. In Greek antiquity the phallus is not represented by an organ but as an insignia; it is the ultimate significative object, which appears when all the veils are lifted. Everything related to it is an object of amputations and interdictions. . . . The phallus represents the intrusion of vital thrusting or growth as such, as what cannot enter the domain of the signifier without being *barred* from it, that is to say, covered over by castration. . . . It is at the level of the Other, in the place where castration manifests itself in the Other, it is in the mother—for both girls and boys—that what is called the castration complex is instituted. It is the desire of the Other which is marked by the bar. [Seminar of April–June, 1958, "Les formations de l'inconscient," *Bulletin de psychologie*, Vol. XII (December 1958), pp. 250–56.]

REJECTION (*forclusion*)
[p. 98]
Lacan has brought out Freud's distinction between the concept of *Verwerfung* ("rejection," "repudiation," "censure"), which he now translates *"forclusion,"* and that of "normal" neurotic repression or *Verdrängung*. In 1954 he translated it *"retranchement"* ("cutting off," "cutting out," "withdrawal") and spoke of the repression of a specific signifier (Freud's Signorelli) as "une parole retranchée" ("Introduction au commentaire de J. Hyppolite" [*Écrits*, p. 369]). In relation to the concept of *béance*, it is worth noting the various meanings of the verb *verwerfen* (basically: "throw away," "throw in the wrong direction," "reject"), especially the reflexive forms meaning "to become warped," "to show a (geological) fault," *Verwerfung* itself also meaning "fault" in this sense. . . . The concept of *Verwerfung* is further referred as "a primordial deficiency [*carence*] in the signifier." [Seminar of January 1958, "Les Formations de l'inconscient," *Bulletin de Psychologie*, Vol. XII (November 1958), pp. 182–92.]
[p. 277]
The notion of *Verwerfung* springs from Freud's use of the term in the Wolf Man's "rejection (repudiation) of castration in the sense of repression" —and as Lacan notes in the *Discours* [*Écrits*, p. 237], the Wolf Man did eventually become psychotic. From the terminological point of view, the notion of *Verwerfung* is to be related to the more strictly discursive term *Verleugnung* (disavowal), which is that upon which Freud relies in his discussion of the psychoses after about 1923. The idea is sometimes expressed as a "withdrawal of cathexis [*Besetzung*] from reality," related to the so-called loss of reality in psychosis. *Verleugnung* is central to his remarks on fetishism (1927)—which, as a perversion, is closer to psychosis than neurosis—where he makes the distinction between "repression" (*Verdrängung*) and "disavowal" (of castration). That his views depend upon an interpretation or value judgment—the castration complex—as well as upon observation, does not of course necessarily invalidate their more general application, especially since the concept of repudiation is intimately connected

with the function of judgment itself in his metapsychological article of 1925 on the *Verneinung*. Lacan, as I have noted, relates the whole question to the phallus, the partial object, castration, and frustration.
[p. 280]
Verwerfung, as a form of negation, consists therefore in *not* symbolizing what should have been symbolized—castration, in the case of the Wolf Man. . . . "The *Verwerfung* therefore cut short any manifestation of the Symbolic order."

REPRESSION *(refoulement)*
[p. 142]
Psychoanalytic "repression" *(Verdrängung)* is rendered by the French *refoulement; répression* in French, best translated "suppression," or "conscious repression," corresponds to the Freudian *Unterdrückung.* There is the further distinction between what Freud called the "primal repression" *(refoulement originaire: Urverdrängung)* and what he first called *Nachdrängen* ("after pressure") and referred to as "repression proper" . . . , later *Nachverdrängung (refoulement après coup:* "after repression"). . . . But for there to be a primal repression, a "mythical" earlier stage must be supposed; for Freud, the primal repression is inaccessible to consciousness; moreover, it never was "conscious." . . . The reader will note the relationship between these concepts and the theory of deferred action *(Nachträglichkeit).*

SIGNIFIER *(signifiant)*
[p. 111]
"The dream-work follows the laws of the signifier." "The unconscious is not the primordial, nor the instinctual, and elementarily it is acquainted only with the elements of the signifier." [Lacan, "L'Instance de la lettre dans l'inconscient ou la raison depuis Freud," *Écrits,* pp. 493–531.] As Lacan points out elsewhere, the dream is not the unconscious, but rather what Freud called the "royal road" to the unconscious, the latter being revealed not by the manifest text of the dream as such, but by the *lacunae* latent within it.
[p. 144]
For Lacan the *signifier* seems to take over the role of the *sign* for Saussure or for Lévi-Strauss. The further Lacan pursues his epistemology of the signifier, the less one hears about the signified (Saussure's "concept") as such.

SUBJECT *(sujet)*
[pp. 141–42]
   The subject . . . begins the analysis by talking about him[self] without talking to *you,* or by talking about him[self]. When he can talk to you

278

about him[self], the analysis will be over. [Lacan, "Introduction au commentaire de Jean Hyppolite sur la *Verneinung* chez Freud," *Écrits,* pp. 369–81.]

What the subject who is speaking says, however empty his discourse may be at first, takes on its effect from the process of approaching to the Word which is realized in his discourse, a coming closer to the Word into which he will fully convert the Truth which his symptoms express [that is, the *parole vide* will become a *parole pleine*]. [*Ibid.*]

[p. 183]

. . . for Lacan, the conscious *cogito* is supplemented by an unconscious subject who may be the subject saying "I think" or "I am," but never both at once, since the question of the subject's being is posed at the level of the unconscious.

[pp. xi–xii]

In 1951 . . . at the Congrès des psychanalystes de langue romane, reacting against an attempt by a colleague to view the transference in terms of Gestalt psychology, Lacan intervened in order to insist upon a dialectical view of the relationship of the analyst and patient. The psychoanalytical experience, he said, "runs its course entirely in a relationship of subject to subject, signifying in effect that it retains a dimension which is irreducible to any psychology considered as an objectification of certain properties of the individual." [*Écrits,* p. 216.] The dialectics of analysis, he continues, are to be found in Freud's experiences of his own countertransference in the case of Dora, a subject to which Lacan returns in the *Discours.** . . . The transference, said Lacan, should surely therefore be considered "as an entity entirely relative to the countertransference defined as the sum of the prejudices, the passions, the embarrassments, even the analyst's insufficient information at this or that moment of the dialectical process." "In other words, the transference involves nothing real in the subject except the appearance of the permanent modes according to which it constitutes its objects, in a moment of stagnation of the dialectic of the analysis." [*Écrits,* p. 225.]

UNCONSCIOUS (*inconscient*)

[p. 144]

For this revelation of meaning [in the practice of analysis] requires that the subject be already ready to hear it—that is to say, that he would not be waiting for it if he had not already found it. But if his comprehension requires the echo of your word, is it not that it is in a Word, which from the fact of being addressed to you was already yours, that the message

---

* The "Discours de Rome": "Fonction et champ de la parole et du langage en psychanalyse," *Écrits,* pp. 237–323.

which he is to receive from it is constituted? Thus the act of the Word appears less as communication than as the grounding of the subjects in an essential annunciation. [Lacan, "Fonction et champ de la parole et du langage en psychanalyse," *Écrits*, pp. 237–323.]

Later, in the formal discussion in 1953, Lacan gave what he called "the general equation of transsubjective communication": "This formula is as follows: the action of the Word, as far as the subject means to ground himself in it, is such that the sender, in order to communicate his message, must receive it from the receiver, and all the same he only manages to do it by emitting his message in an inverted form." [*Ibid.*]

The unconscious is that discourse of the Other where the subject receives in the inverted form suited to the promise, his own forgotten message. [Lacan, "La Psychanalyse et son enseignement," *Écrits,* pp. 437–59.]

WORD (*parole*)
[pp. 115–16]

Symptoms of conversion, inhibition, anguish, these are not there to offer you the opportunity to confirm their nodal points, however seductive their topology may be; it is a question of untying these knots, and this means to return them to the Word function that they hold in a discourse whose signification determines their use and their sense. [Lacan, "Fonction et champ de la parole et du langage en psychanalyse," *Écrits,* pp. 237–323.]

The letter of the message is the important thing here. In order to grasp it, one must stop an instant at the fundamentally equivocal character of the Word, insofar as its function is as much to hide as to uncover. . . . It is this [division into the different parts of an] orchestral score inherent in the ambiguity of Language which alone explains the multiplicity of the ways of access to the secret of the Word. The fact remains that there is only one text where it is possible to read what the Word says and what it does not say, and that it is to this text that the symptoms are connected just as intimately as is a rebus to the sentence it represents.

For some time now there has been utter confusion between the multiple ways of access to the deciphering of this sentence, and what Freud calls the overdetermination of the symptoms which represent it. [*Ibid.*]

Subject Index

aggression (aggressiveness), 11, 25–26, 68, 88, 103, 111, 158
anxiety: persecution, 5, 11, 89; phobic, 7, 66–70, 148–78; hypochondriac, 56; parental, 70–2, 80–1, 131–6, 188–9

behaviorism, 12, 23

castration fears, 8, 39, 64, 135, 165, 166, 190, 199, 219, 221
child analysis: *see* psychoanalysis, of children
child guidance movement, 54
childhood: reconstructions of, 3–4, 14; conflicts of, 23; studies of, 24
communication: as collective process, 3, 96, 194, 200; problem of, 42–4; symptomatic, 57–8, 61; closed-circuit, 118, 125–6, 127; of drama, 119; between normal and retarded, 205; *see also* language; symptom condensation, 78 *n.*
conflict, 23–6; *see also* childhood
countertransference, 4, 48, 97, 120, 226
cure, psychoanalytic, 33, 53, 125, 126; *see also* psychoanalysis, of children

daydreaming, 53, 205
death: theme of, in the case of Sam, 34–42; in the case of Emile, 74–7; as "key" signifier, 79, *n.*, 150, 151;

in the case of Guy, 159, 160–1, 162–3; in the case of Emmanuel, 219
debility, pseudo-, 63
defense mechanisms, 18, 118, 189
deficit, organic, 72, 78; *see also* organicity
demands, 56, 59, 64, 96, 121, 122, 148, 149, 194, 195
dementia praecox, 100, 126
deprivation, parental, 15; *see also* parents, and child's illness
desire, 9 *n.,* 39, 56–7, 96, 121, 122, 149, 165, 184, 220; language of, 12, 136; responses to, 28; of the Other, 33, 42, 44, 46, 50, 60, 83, 98, 115, 122, 166, 167, 176, 190; *see also* subject
development: current theories of, 45, 206; stages in, 48
displacement, 78 *n.*
doctor-patient relationship, 204
"Dreams and Occultism" (Freud), 42

éducateur, in France, 224 *n.*
ego-ideal, 14–15, 118; *see also* identity
encephalopathy, 72, 116
Externat Médico-pédagogique (special school for mentally retarded children), 224 *n.;* experiment in, 226–42; purpose of, 240–2

281

Index of Case Histories

Index of Authors

Abraham, Karl, 6, 11, 110, 126
Ackerman, Nathan W., 197 *n.*
Amado, Georges, 228
Anzieu, Didier, 226 *n.*
Aubrey, Jenny, 136 *n.*
Aulagnier, Piera, 103 *n.*, 123 *n.*, 194 *n.*, 195 *n.*

Bargues, Raymonde, 136 *n.*
Binswanger, Ludwig, 12
Bleuler, Eugen, 100, 126
Bleuler, Manfred, 100
Burlingham, Dorothy, 7, 55
Buxbaum, Edith, 54 *n.*

Danos, J., 224 *n.*
Daumezon, G., 226
Debacker, F., 4–5
Decroly, Ovide, 206
Diatkine, R., 101 *n.*
Dolto, Françoise, 24–6, 27 *n.*

Erikson, Erik H., 14–15, 18, 34–42, 45, 46, 47, 198
Esquirol, J.-E.-T., 203
Esterson, Aaron, 101 *n.*, 198, 242 *n.*

Faergeman, Poul Martin, 100 *n.*
Ferenczi, Sandor, 85 *n.*
Foucault, Michel, 204
Fraiberg, Selma, 63 *n.*
Freud, Anna, 6, 7, 11, 17, 54

Freud, Sigmund, 3–20 *passim,* 23–4, 29, 31–2, 33, 40, 42–5, 53, 57 *n.*, 59, 77–8, 79, 83, 84 *n.*, 97–8, 110, 111, 126, 193, 198, 204, 206, 251

Goldberger, Alice, 55 *n.*
Green, André, 124 *n.*
Grinberg, Léon, 95 *n.*

Haworth, Mary R., 18 *n.*
Hellman, Ilse, 43 *n.*, 56
Hug-Hellmuth, H., 4, 6, 7

Itard, Jean, 206–9

Klein, Melanie, 6–7, 10–12, 19, 41 *n.*, 98, 103, 110, 120 *n.*, 158, 196, 238
Kraepelin, Emil, 100, 126
Kut, Sara, 63 *n.*

Lacan, Jacques, 10 *n.*, 11, 14 *n.*, 15, 19 *n.*, 23 n., 41, 46, 51 *n.*, 53 *n.*, 57 *n.*, 59, 60 n., 62, 78 *n.*, 96, 98, 101, 106, 108 *n.*, 121 *n.*, 122, 193 *n.*, 199 *n.*
Laing, R. D., 12–14, 101–2, 198, 242 *n.*
Lang, J.-L., 101
Laplanche, Jean, 78 *n.*
Lebo, Dell, 18 *n.*
Lebovici, Serge, 47 *n.*, 48 *n.*
Leclaire, Serge, 78 *n.*, 108 *n.*

285